THE

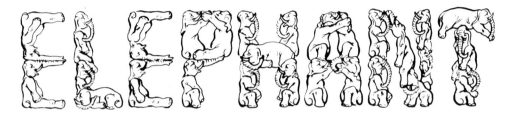

BOOK

Dennis Pepper

Oxford University Press 1983
Oxford   Toronto   Melbourne

Oxford University Press, Walton Street, Oxford OX2 6DP

Oxford London Glasgow
New York Toronto Melbourne Auckland
Kuala Lumpur Singapore Hong Kong Tokyo
Delhi Bombay Calcutta Madras Karachi
Nairobi Dar es Salaam Cape Town

and associated companies in
Beirut Berlin Ibadan Mexico City Nicosia

Oxford is a trade mark of Oxford University Press
This selection © Dennis Pepper 1983

British Library Cataloguing in Publication Data

The Elephant book.
 1. Elephants—Juvenile literature
 I. Pepper, Dennis
 599.6'1   QL737.P98

 ISBN 0-19-278100-6

Phototypeset by Tradespools Limited, Frome, Somerset, in Trump (Medieval).
What else could we use in the Elephant Book?
Printed in Hong Kong

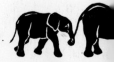

Contents

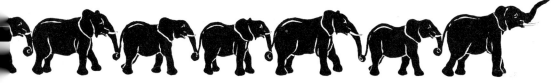

Elephant, who brings death.
Elephant, a spirit in the bush.
With a single hand
he can pull two palm trees to the ground.
If he had two hands
he would tear the sky like an old rag.
The spirit who eats dog,
the spirit who eats ram,
the spirit who eats
a whole palm fruit with its thorns.
With his four mortar legs
he tramples down the grass.
Wherever he walks
the grass is forbidden to stand again.

Yoruba song

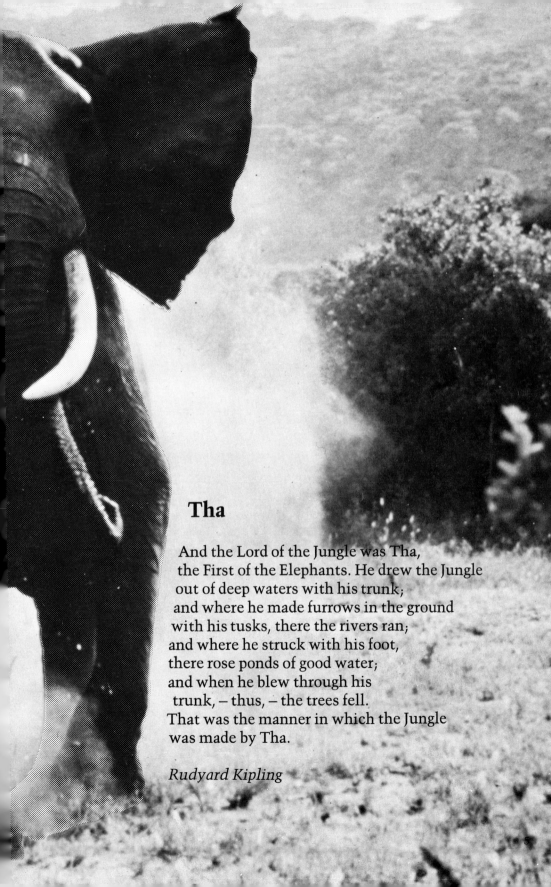

Tha

And the Lord of the Jungle was Tha,
  the First of the Elephants. He drew the Jungle
  out of deep waters with his trunk;
  and where he made furrows in the ground
  with his tusks, there the rivers ran;
  and where he struck with his foot,
  there rose ponds of good water;
  and when he blew through his
  trunk, – thus, – the trees fell.
That was the manner in which the Jungle
  was made by Tha.

Rudyard Kipling

How the Elephant Became

The unhappiest of all the creatures was Bombo. Bombo didn't know what to become. At one time he thought he might make a fairly good horse. At another time he thought that perhaps he was meant to be a kind of bull. But it was no good. Not only the horses, but all the other creatures too, gathered to laugh at him when he tried to be a horse. And when he tried to be a bull, the bulls just walked away shaking their heads.

'Be yourself,' they all said.

Bombo sighed. That's all he ever heard: 'Be yourself. Be yourself.' What was himself? That's what he wanted to know.

So most of the time he just stood, with sad eyes, letting the wind blow his ears this way and that, while the other creatures raced around him and above him, perfecting themselves.

'I'm just stupid,' he said to himself. 'Just stupid and slow and I shall never become anything.'

That was his main trouble, he felt sure. He was much too slow and clumsy – and so big! None of the other creatures were anywhere near so big. He searched hard to find another creature as big as he was, but there was not one. This made him feel all the more silly and in the way.

But this was not all. He had great ears that flapped and hung, and a long, long nose. His nose was useful. He could pick things up with it. But none of the other creatures had a nose anything like it. They all had small neat noses, and they laughed at his. In fact, with that, and his ears, and his long white sticking-out tusks, he was a sight.

As he stood, there was a sudden thunder of hooves. Bombo looked up in alarm.

'Aside, aside, aside!' roared a huge voice. 'We're going down to drink.'

Bombo managed to force his way backwards into a painful clump of thorn-bushes, just in time to let Buffalo charge past with all his family. Their long black bodies shone, their curved horns tossed, their tails screwed and curled, as they pounded down towards the water in a cloud of dust. The earth shook under them.

'There's no doubt,' said Bombo, 'who they are.
If only I could be as sure of what I am
as Buffalo is of what he is.'
Then he pulled himself together.
'To be myself,' he said aloud,
'I shall have to do something
that no other creature does.
Lion roars and pounces, and
Buffalo charges up and down bellowing.
Each of these creatures does something
that no other creature does. So.
What shall I do?'

He thought hard for a minute.

Then he lay down,
rolled over on to his back, and waved his
four great legs in the air.

After that he stood on his head and
lifted his hind legs straight up
as if he were going to sunburn
the soles of his feet.

From this position, he lowered himself
back on to his four feet, stood up and looked round.

The others should soon get to know
me by that, he thought.

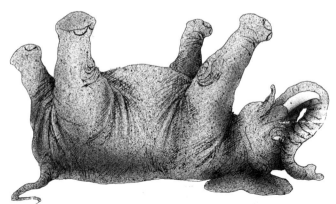

Nobody was in sight, so he waited until a pack of wolves appeared on the horizon. Then he began again. On to his back, his legs in the air, then on to his head, and his hind legs straight up.

'Phew!' he grunted, as he lowered himself. 'I shall need some practice before I can keep this up for long.'

When he stood up and looked round him this second time, he got a shock. All the animals were round him in a ring, rolling on their sides with laughter.

'Do it again! Oh, do it again!' they were crying, as they rolled and laughed. 'Do it again. Oh, I shall die with laughter. Oh, my sides, my sides!'

Bombo stared at them in horror.

After a few minutes the laughter died down.

'Come on!' roared Lion. 'Do it again and make us laugh. You look so silly when you do it.'

But Bombo just stood. This was much worse than imitating some other animal. He had never made them laugh so much before.

He sat down and pretended to be inspecting one of his feet, as if he were alone. And, one by one, now that there was nothing to laugh at, the other animals walked away, still chuckling over what they had seen.

'Next show same time tomorrow!' shouted Fox, and they all burst out laughing again.

Bombo sat, playing with his foot, letting the tears trickle down his long nose.

Well, he'd had enough. He'd tried to be himself, and all the animals had laughed at him.

That night he waded out to a small island in the middle of the great river that ran through the forest. And there, from then on, Bombo lived alone, seen by nobody but the little birds and a few beetles.

One night, many years later, Parrot suddenly screamed and flew up into the air above the trees. All his feathers were singed. The forest was on fire.

Within a few minutes, the animals were running for their lives. Jaguar, Wolf, Stag, Cow, Bear, Sheep, Cockerel, Mouse, Giraffe – all were running side by side and jumping over each other to get away from the flames. Behind them, the fire came through the treetops like a terrific red wind.

'Oh dear! Oh dear! Our houses, our children!' cried the animals.

Lion and Buffalo were running along with the rest.

'The fire will go as far as the forest goes, and the forest goes on for ever,' they cried, and ran with sparks falling into their hair. On and on they ran, hour after hour, and all they could hear was the thunder of the fire at their tails.

On into the middle of the next day, and still they were running.

At last they came to the wide, deep, swift river. They could go no farther. Behind them the fire boomed as it leapt from tree to tree. Smoke lay so thickly over the forest and the river that the sun could not be seen. The animals floundered in the shallows at the river's edge, trampling the banks to mud, treading on each other, coughing and sneezing in the white ashes that were falling thicker than thick snow out of the cloud of smoke. Fox sat on Sheep and Sheep sat on Rhinoceros.

They all set up a terrible roaring, wailing, crying, howling, moaning sound. It seemed like the end of the animals. The fire came nearer, bending over them like a thundering roof, while the black river swirled and rumbled beside them.

Out on his island stood Bombo, admiring the fire which made a fine sight through the smoke with its high spikes of red flame. He knew he was quite safe on his island. The fire couldn't cross that great stretch of water very easily.

At first he didn't see the animals crowding low by the edge of the water. The smoke and ash were too thick in the air. But soon he heard them. Hè recognized Lion's voice shouting:

'Keep ducking yourselves in the water. Keep your fur wet and the sparks will not burn you.'

And the voice of Sheep crying:

'If we duck ourselves we're swept away by the river.'

And the other creatures – Gnu, Ferret, Cobra, Partridge, crying:

'We must drown or burn. Good-bye, brothers and sisters!'

It certainly did seem like the end of the animals.

Without a pause, Bombo pushed his way into the water. The river was deep, the current heavy and fierce, but Bombo's legs were both long and strong. Burnt trees, that had fallen into the river higher up and were drifting down, banged against him, but he hardly felt them.

In a few minutes he was coming up into shallow water towards the animals. He was almost too late. The flames were forcing them, step by step, into the river, where the current was snatching them away.

Lion was sitting on Buffalo, Wolf was sitting on Lion, Wildcat on Wolf, Badger on Wildcat, Cockerel on Badger, Rat on Cockerel, Weasel on Rat, Lizard on Weasel, Tree-Creeper on Lizard, Harvest Mouse on Tree-Creeper, Beetle on Harvest Mouse, Wasp on Beetle, and on top of Wasp, Ant, gazing at the raging flames through his spectacles and covering his ears from their roar.

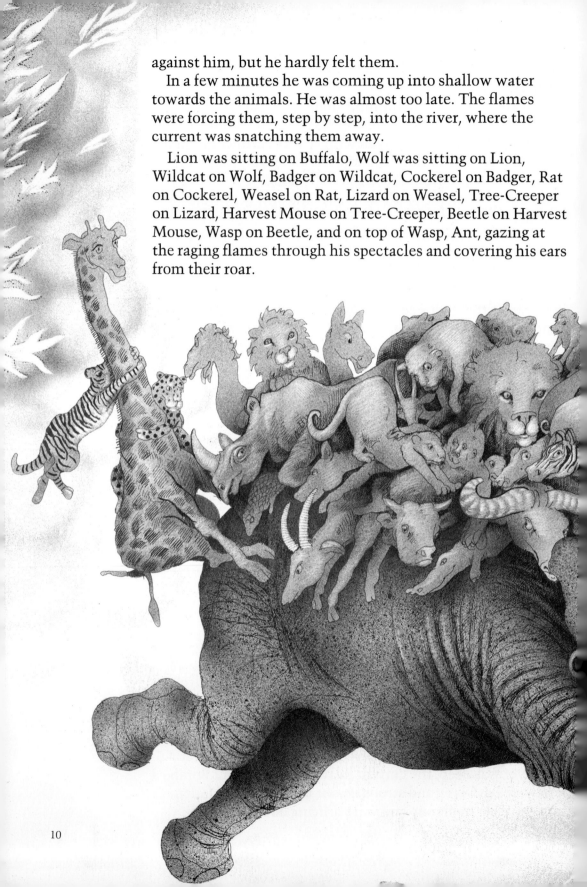

When the animals saw Bombo looming through the smoke, a great shout went up:

'It's Bombo! It's Bombo!'

All the animals took up the cry:

'Bombo! Bombo!'

Bombo kept coming closer. As he came, he sucked up water in his long silly nose and squirted it over his back, to protect himself from the heat and the sparks. Then, with the same long, silly nose he reached out and began to pick up the animals, one by one, and seat them on his back.

'Take us!' cried Mole.

'Take us!' cried Monkey.

He loaded his back with the creatures that had hooves and big feet; then he told the little clinging things to cling on to the great folds of his ears. Soon he had every single creature aboard. Then he turned and began to wade back across the river, carrying all the animals of the forest towards safety.

Once they were safe on the island they danced for joy.

Then they sat down to watch the fire.

Suddenly Mouse gave a shout:

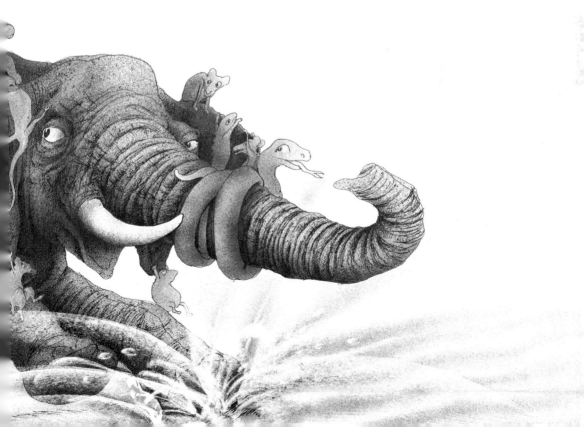

'Look! The wind is bringing the sparks across the river. The sparks are blowing into the island trees. We shall burn here too.'

As he spoke, one of the trees on the edge of the island crackled into flames. The animals set up a great cry and began to run in all directions.

'Help! Help! Help! We shall burn here too!'

But Bombo was ready. He put those long silly tusks of his, that he had once been so ashamed of, under the roots of the burning tree and heaved it into the river. He threw every tree into the river till the island was bare. The sparks now fell on to the bare torn ground, where the animals trod them out easily. Bombo had saved them again.

Next morning the fire had died out at the river's edge. The animals on the island looked across at the smoking, blackened plain where the forest had been. Then they looked round for Bombo.

He was nowhere to be seen.

'Bombo!' they shouted. 'Bombo!' And listened to the echo. But he had gone.

He is still very hard to find. Though he is huge and strong, he is very quiet.

But what did become of him in the end? Where is he now?

Ask any of the animals, and they will tell you:

'Though he is shy, he is the strongest, the cleverest, and the kindest of all the animals. He can carry anything and he can push anything down. He can pick you up in his nose and wave you in the air. We would make him our king if we could get him to wear a crown.'

Ted Hughes

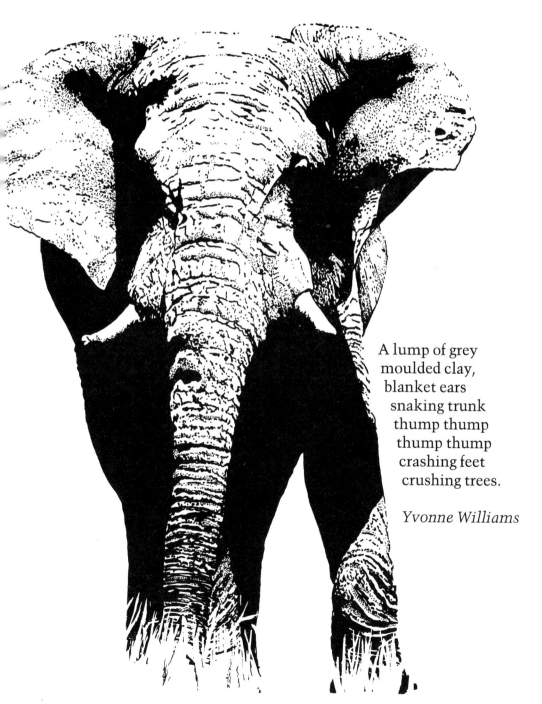

A lump of grey
moulded clay,
blanket ears
snaking trunk
thump thump
thump thump
crashing feet
crushing trees.

Yvonne Williams

Mouse and the Elephant

Once there was a rogue elephant. He smashed through the jungle tearing up the trees and throwing them about. He was big and strong and he trumpeted loudly for all the animals to hear.

As he went on his way he noticed a small mouse cowering down by the side of a tree.

'HA!' he roared. 'YOU COULDN'T DO THAT!'

'N-no, I couldn't,' squeaked the mouse. 'I've been very poorly.'

– Baby elephants.

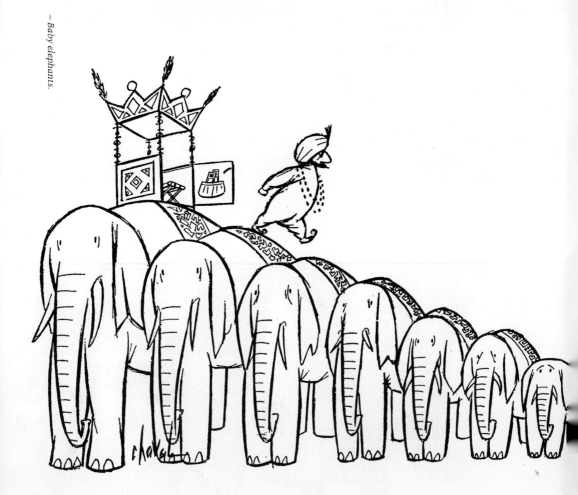

Why Elephants don't Fly

Long long ago elephants used to fly. They had great wings. One day an elephant went down to a lake to drink water. There was a crocodile in the lake and when it heard the elephant splashing about, it wondered what this great creature was. It swam through the water and caught it by the leg.

The elephant tried to fly away but could not because of the crocodile, which dragged it into deep water. They struggled together for twelve years and thirteen ages until the elephant called on Bhagavan for help.

Bhagavan came and saw that the crocodile had torn the wings of the elephant and that the creature was worn out and about to die. Its whole body was sunk under the water except for its nose and ears. Bhagavan pulled the nose and it became very long; he took it by the ears and they became very broad.

Then he cut off what was left of the wings, for elephants were always coming down from the skies and crashing on houses and cowsheds and ruining them.

So Bhagavan said, 'From now on elephants shall not fly.'

Indian story

What do you call an elephant that flies?

– A jumbo jet.

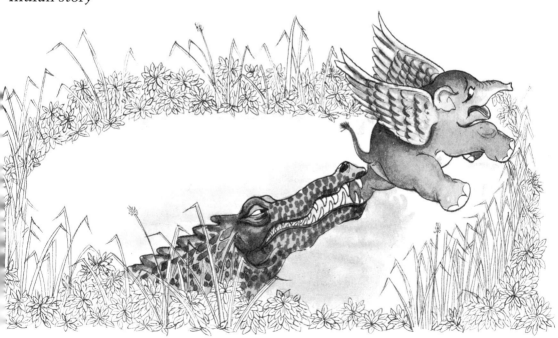

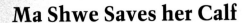

Ma Shwe Saves her Calf

One evening, when the Upper Taungdwin River was in heavy spate, I was listening and hoping to hear the boom and roar of timber coming from upstream. Directly below my camp the banks of the river were steep and rocky and twelve to fifteen feet high. About fifty yards away on the other side, the bank was made up of ledges of shale strata. Although it was already nearly dusk, by watching these ledges being successively submerged, I was trying to judge how fast the water was rising.

I was suddenly alarmed by hearing an elephant roaring as though frightened, and, looking down, I saw three or four men rushing up and down on the opposite bank in a state of great excitement. I realized at once that something was wrong, and ran down to the edge of the near bank and there saw Ma Shwe with her three-months-old calf, trapped in the fast-rising torrent. She herself was still in her depth, as the water was about six feet deep. But there was a life-and-death struggle going on. Her calf was screaming with terror and was afloat like a cork. Ma Shwe was as near to the far bank as she could get, holding her whole body against the raging and increasing torrent, and keeping the calf pressed against her massive body. Every now and then the swirling water would sweep the calf away; then, with terrific strength, she would encircle it with her trunk and pull it upstream to rest against her body again.

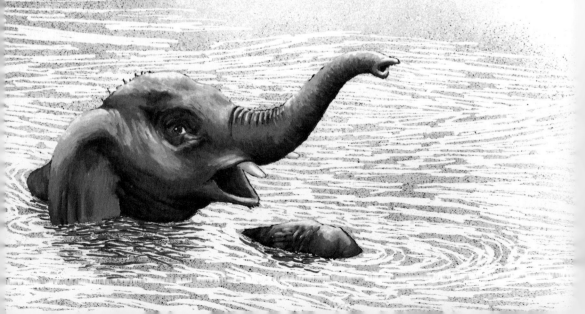

There was a sudden rise in the water, as if a two-foot bore had come down, and the calf was washed clean over the mother's hindquarters and was gone. She turned to chase it, like an otter after a fish, but she had travelled about fifty yards downstream and, plunging and sometimes afloat, had crossed to my side of the river, before she had caught up with it and got it back. For what seemed minutes, she pinned the calf with her head and trunk against the rocky bank. Then, with a really gigantic effort, she picked it up in her trunk and reared up until she was half standing on her hind legs, so as to be able to place it on a narrow shelf of rock, five feet above the flood level.

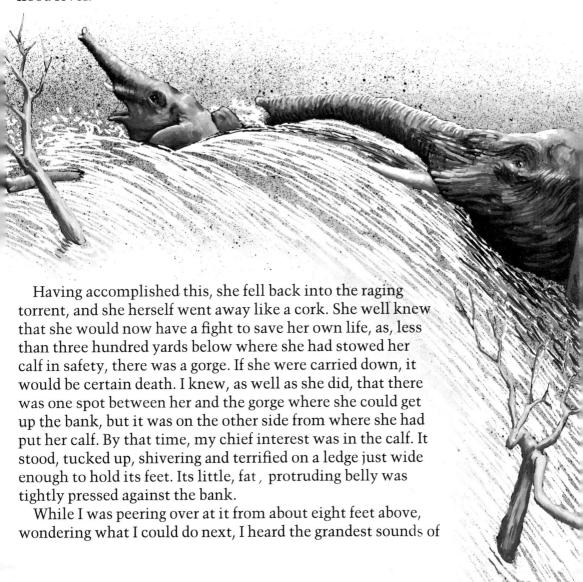

Having accomplished this, she fell back into the raging torrent, and she herself went away like a cork. She well knew that she would now have a fight to save her own life, as, less than three hundred yards below where she had stowed her calf in safety, there was a gorge. If she were carried down, it would be certain death. I knew, as well as she did, that there was one spot between her and the gorge where she could get up the bank, but it was on the other side from where she had put her calf. By that time, my chief interest was in the calf. It stood, tucked up, shivering and terrified on a ledge just wide enough to hold its feet. Its little, fat, protruding belly was tightly pressed against the bank.

While I was peering over at it from about eight feet above, wondering what I could do next, I heard the grandest sounds of a mother's love I can remember. Ma Shwe had crossed the river and got up the bank, and was making her way back as fast as she could, calling the whole time – a defiant roar, but to her calf it was music. The two little ears, like little maps of India, were cocked forward, listening to the only sound that mattered, the call of her mother.

Any wild schemes which had raced through my head of recovering the calf by ropes disappeared as fast as I had formed them, when I saw Ma Shwe emerge from the jungle and appear on the opposite bank. When she saw her calf, she stopped roaring and began rumbling, a never-to-be-forgotten sound, not unlike that made by a very high-powered car when accelerating. It is the sound of pleasure, like a cat's purring, and delighted she must have been to see her calf still in the same spot, where she had put her half an hour before.

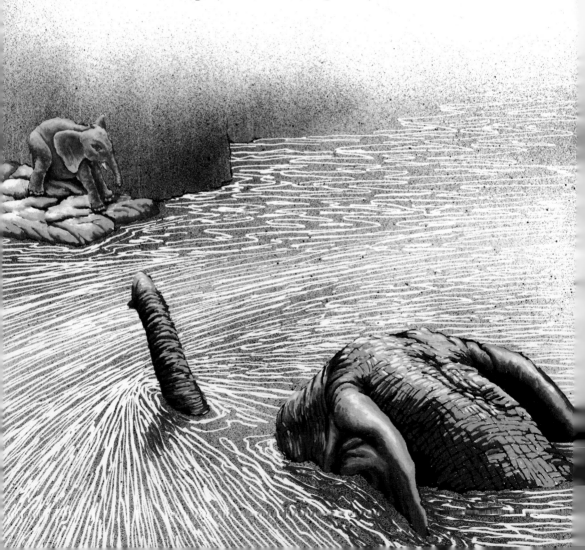

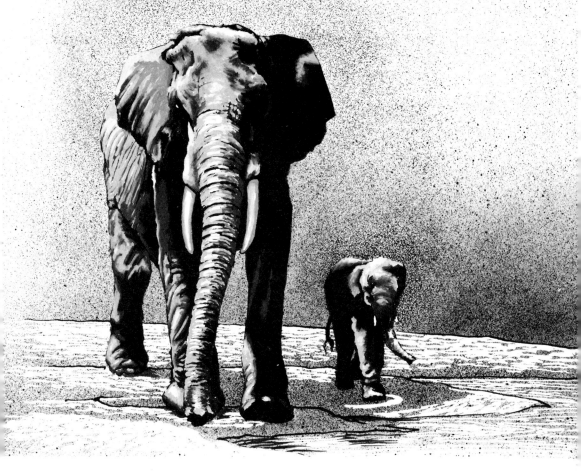

As darkness fell, the muffled boom of floating logs hitting against each other came from upstream. A torrential rain was falling, and the river still separated the mother and her calf. I decided that I could do nothing but wait and see what happened. Twice before turning in for the night I went down to the bank and picked out the calf with my torch, but this seemed to disturb it, so I went away.

It was just as well I did, because at dawn Ma Shwe and her calf were together – both on the far bank. The spate had subsided to a mere foot of dirty-coloured water. No one in the camp had seen Ma Shwe recover her calf, but she must have lifted it down from the ledge in the same way as she had put it there.

Five years later, when the calf came to be named, the Burmans christened it Ma Yay Yee (Miss Laughing Water).

J. H. Williams

The Big Drought

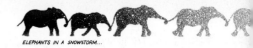

ELEPHANTS IN A SNOWSTORM...

Once there was a big drought over the land. The only water left was in a small pool where the antelopes came to drink. When the leader of the elephants found the pool he drove the antelopes away so that the elephants could have it to themselves.

'This can't go on,' thought the oldest and wisest of the antelopes. 'Soon the water will have gone and we shall all die.' So he climbed a hill by the side of the trail and waited for the leader of the elephants to pass.

'O Great King of the Elephants!' he cried as the elephant leader came into sight. 'I come to you with a message from the Monarch of the Moon.'

'What's that?' said the elephant. 'Who are you? What do you want?'

'I am the Moon King's special messenger,' said the antelope, 'and I come to you by his command. You have driven his guardians from his Sacred Pool and he is very angry. Tonight he will punish you.'

'Oh,' said the elephant. 'I'm very sorry. I didn't know. We won't go near the pool again.'

'Sorrow comes too late,' said the antelope. 'If you would escape punishment and live in peace, you must come to the Sacred Pool tonight and ask the Moon King's forgiveness.'

That night the anxious elephant came to the pool. The special messenger showed him the Moon King's reflection quivering in the water and ordered him to kneel.

'Great King,' said the elephant in a tiny voice, 'I am very sorry. Though my offence is great, it was done in ignorance. Grant me forgiveness, great King, and I will take my people far away.'

At that moment clouds covered the moon.

'It is a sign,' said the antelope quickly. 'Go now before my master changes his mind.'

'And don't come back!' he shouted after the elephant's disappearing tail.

After that the antelopes had the pool to themselves.

Hitopadesha

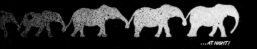

...AT NIGHT!

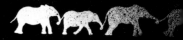

Way Down South

Way down South where bananas grow,
A grasshopper stepped on an elephant's toe.
The elephant said, with tears in his eyes,
'Pick on somebody your own size.'

Traditional American

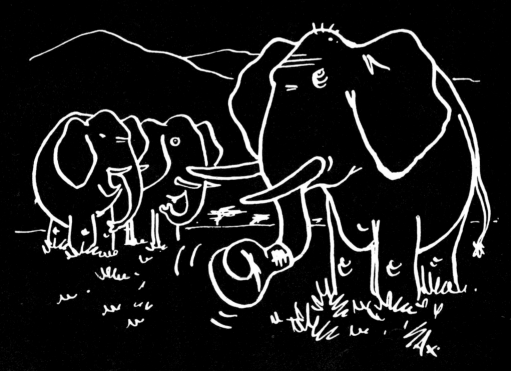

'HE'S IN A NASTY MOOD TODAY!'

The Elephant's Child

In the High and Far-Off Times the Elephant, O Best Beloved, had no trunk. He had only a blackish, bulgy nose, as big as a boot, that he could wriggle about from side to side; but he couldn't pick up things with it. But there was one Elephant – a new Elephant – an Elephant's Child – who was full of 'satiable curtiosity, and that means he asked ever so many questions. *And* he lived in Africa, and he filled all Africa with his 'satiable curtiosities. He asked his tall aunt, the Ostrich, why her tail-feathers grew just so, and his tall aunt, the Ostrich, spanked him with her hard, hard claw. He asked his tall uncle, the Giraffe, what made his skin spotty, and his tall uncle, the Giraffe, spanked him with his hard, hard hoof. And still he was full of 'satiable curtiosity! He asked his broad aunt, the Hippopotamus, why her eyes were red, and his broad aunt, the Hippopotamus, spanked him with her broad, broad hoof; and he asked his hairy uncle, the Baboon, why melons tasted just so, and his hairy uncle, the Baboon, spanked him with his hairy, hairy paw. And *still* he was full of 'satiable curtiosity! He asked questions about everything that he saw, or heard, or felt, or smelt, or touched, and all his uncles and his aunts spanked him. And still he was full of 'satiable curtiosity!

One fine morning this 'satiable Elephant's Child asked a new fine question that he had never asked before. He asked, 'What does the Crocodile have for dinner?' Then everybody said, 'Hush!' in a loud and dretful tone, and they spanked him immediately and directly, without stopping, for a long time.

By and by, when that was finished, he came upon Kolokolo Bird sitting in the middle of a wait-a-bit thorn-bush, and he said, 'My father has spanked me, and my mother has spanked me; all my aunts and uncles have spanked me for my 'satiable curtiosity; and *still* I want to know what the Crocodile has for dinner!'

Then Kolokolo Bird said, with a mournful cry, 'Go to the banks of the great grey-green, greasy Limpopo River, all set about with fever-trees, and find out.'

That very next morning, this 'satiable Elephant's Child took a hundred pounds of bananas (the little short red kind), and a hundred pounds of sugar-cane (the long purple kind),

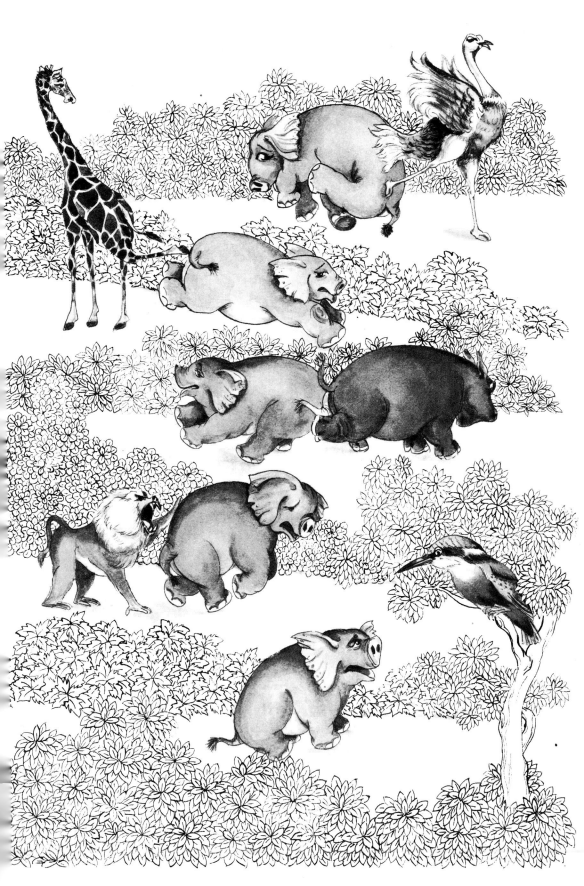

and seventeen melons (the greeny-crackly kind), and said to all his dear families, 'Good-bye. I am going to the great grey-green, greasy Limpopo River, all set about with fever trees, to find out what the Crocodile has for dinner.' And they all spanked him once more for luck, though he asked them most politely to stop.

Then he went away, a little warm, but not at all astonished, eating melons, and throwing the rind about, because he could not pick it up.

He went from Graham's Town to Kimberley, and from Kimberley to Khama's Country, and from Khama's Country he went east by north, eating melons all the time, till at last he came to the banks of the great grey-green, greasy Limpopo River, all set about with fever-trees, precisely as Kolokolo Bird had said.

Now you must know and understand, O Best Beloved, that till that very week, and day, and hour, and minute, this 'satiable Elephant's Child had never seen a Crocodile, and did not know what one was like. It was all his 'satiable curtiosity.

The first thing that he found was a Bi-Coloured-Python-Rock-Snake curled round a rock.

''Scuse me,' said the Elephant's Child most politely, 'but have you seen such a thing as a Crocodile in these promiscuous parts?'

'*Have* I seen a Crocodile?' said the Bi-Coloured-Python-Rock-Snake, in a voice of dretful scorn. 'What will you ask me next?'

''Scuse me,' said the Elephant's Child, 'but could you kindly tell me what he has for dinner?'

Then the Bi-Coloured-Python-Rock-Snake uncoiled himself very quickly from the rock, and spanked the Elephant's Child with his scalesome, flailsome tail.

'That is odd,' said the Elephant's Child, 'because my father and my mother, and my uncle and my aunt, not to mention my other aunt, the Hippopotamus, and my other uncle, the Baboon, have all spanked me for my 'satiable curtiosity – and I suppose this is the same thing.'

So he said good-bye very politely to the Bi-Coloured-Python-Rock-Snake, and helped to coil him up on the rock again, and went on, a little warm, but not at all astonished, eating melons, and throwing the rind about, because he could

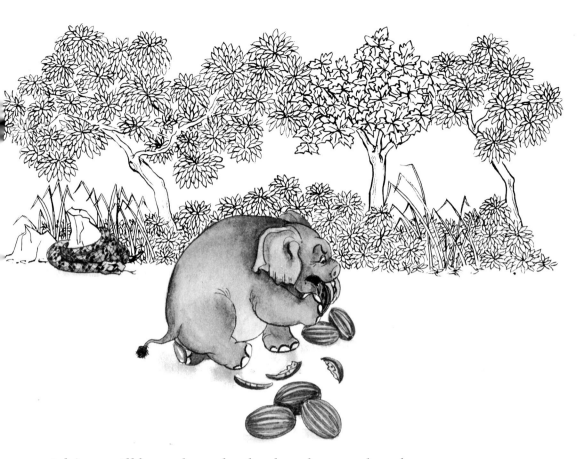

not pick it up, till he trod on what he thought was a log of wood at the very edge of the great grey-green, greasy Limpopo River, all set about with fever-trees.

But it was really the Crocodile, O Best Beloved, and the Crocodile winked one eye – like this!

''Scuse me,' said the Elephant's Child most politely, 'but do you happen to have seen a Crocodile in these promiscuous parts?'

Then the Crocodile winked the other eye, and lifted half his tail out of the mud; and the Elephant's child stepped back most politely, because he did not wish to be spanked again.

'Come hither, Little One,' said the Crocodile. 'Why do you ask such things?'

''Scuse me,' said the Elephant's Child most politely, 'but my father has spanked me, my mother has spanked me, not to mention my tall aunt, the Ostrich, and my tall uncle, the Giraffe, who can kick ever so hard, as well as my broad aunt, the Hippopotamus, and my hairy uncle, the Baboon, *and* including the Bi-Coloured-Python-Rock-Snake, with the scalesome, flailsome tail, just up the bank, who spanks harder

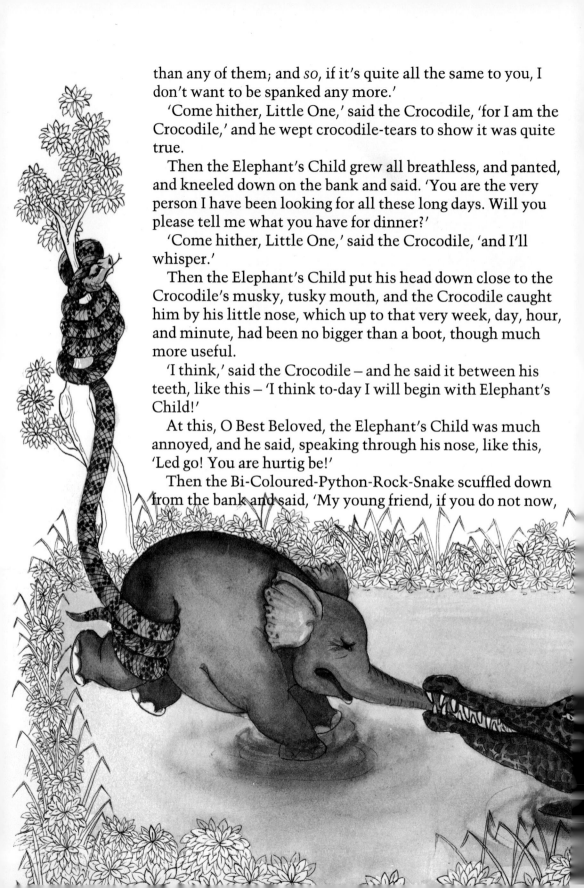

than any of them; and *so*, if it's quite all the same to you, I don't want to be spanked any more.'

'Come hither, Little One,' said the Crocodile, 'for I am the Crocodile,' and he wept crocodile-tears to show it was quite true.

Then the Elephant's Child grew all breathless, and panted, and kneeled down on the bank and said. 'You are the very person I have been looking for all these long days. Will you please tell me what you have for dinner?'

'Come hither, Little One,' said the Crocodile, 'and I'll whisper.'

Then the Elephant's Child put his head down close to the Crocodile's musky, tusky mouth, and the Crocodile caught him by his little nose, which up to that very week, day, hour, and minute, had been no bigger than a boot, though much more useful.

'I think,' said the Crocodile – and he said it between his teeth, like this – 'I think to-day I will begin with Elephant's Child!'

At this, O Best Beloved, the Elephant's Child was much annoyed, and he said, speaking through his nose, like this, 'Led go! You are hurtig be!'

Then the Bi-Coloured-Python-Rock-Snake scuffled down from the bank and said, 'My young friend, if you do not now, immediately and instantly, pull as hard as ever you can, it is my opinion that your acquaintance in the large-pattern leather ulster' (and by this he meant the Crocodile) 'will jerk you into yonder limpid stream before you can say Jack Robinson.'

This is the way Bi-Coloured-Python-Rock-Snakes always talk.

Then the Elephant's Child sat back on his little haunches, and pulled, and pulled, and pulled, and his nose began to stretch. And the Crocodile floundered into the water, making it all creamy with great sweeps of his tail, and *he* pulled, and pulled, and pulled.

And the Elephant's Child's nose kept on stretching; and the Elephant's Child spread all his little four legs and pulled, and pulled, and pulled, and his nose kept on stretching; and the Crocodile threshed his tail like an oar, and *he* pulled, and pulled and pulled, and at each pull the Elephant's Child's nose grew longer and longer – and it hurt him hijjus!

Then the Elephant's Child felt his legs slipping, and he said through his nose, which was now nearly five feet long, 'This is too butch for be!'

Then the Bi-Coloured-Python-Rock-Snake came down from the bank, and knotted himself in a double-clove-hitch round the Elephant's Child's hind-legs, and said, 'Rash and

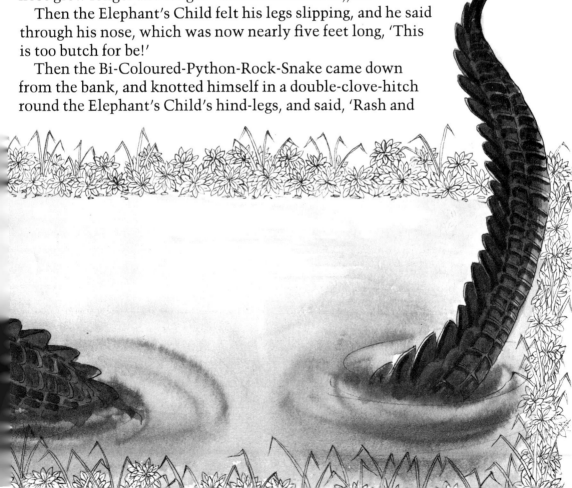

inexperienced traveller, we will now seriously devote ourselves to a little high tension, because if we do not, it is my impression that yonder self-propelling man-of-war with the armour-plated upper deck' (and by this, O Best Beloved, he meant the Crocodile) 'will permanently vitiate your future career.'

That is the way all Bi-Coloured-Python-Rock-Snakes always talk.

So he pulled, and the Elephant's Child pulled, and the Crocodile pulled; but the Elephant's Child and the Bi-Coloured-Python-Rock-Snake pulled hardest; and at last the Crocodile let go of the Elephant's Child's nose with a plop that you could hear all up and down the Limpopo.

Then the Elephant's Child sat down most hard and sudden; but first he was careful to say 'Thank you' to the Bi-Coloured-Python-Rock-Snake; and next he was kind to his poor pulled nose, and wrapped it all up in cool banana leaves, and hung it in the great grey-green, greasy Limpopo to cool.

'What are you doing that for?' said the Bi-Coloured-Python-Rock-Snake.

''Scuse me,' said the Elephant's Child, 'but my nose is badly out of shape, and I am waiting for it to shrink.'

'Then you will have to wait a long time,' said the Bi-Coloured-Python-Rock-Snake. 'Some people do not know what is good for them.'

The Elephant's Child sat there for three days waiting for his nose to shrink. But it never grew any shorter, and, besides, it made him squint. For, O Best Beloved, you will see and understand that the Crocodile had pulled it out into a really truly trunk same as all Elephants have to-day.

At the end of the third day a fly came and stung him on the shoulder, and before he knew what he was doing he lifted up his trunk and hit that fly dead with the end of it.

''Vantage number one!' said the Bi-Coloured-Python-Rock-Snake. 'You couldn't have done that with a mere-smear nose. Try and eat a little now.'

Before he thought what he was doing the Elephant's Child put out his trunk and plucked a large bundle of grass, dusted it clean against his fore-legs, and stuffed it into his own mouth.

''Vantage number two!' said the Bi-Coloured-Python-Rock-

Snake. 'You couldn't have done that with a mere-smear nose. Don't you think the sun is very hot here?'

'It is,' said the Elephant's Child, and before he thought what he was doing he schlooped up a schloop of mud from the banks of the great grey-green, greasy Limpopo, and slapped it on his head, where it made a cool schloopy-sloshy mud-cap all trickly behind his ears.

''Vantage number three!' said the Bi-Coloured-Python-Rock-Snake. 'You couldn't have done that with a mere-smear nose. Now how do you feel about being spanked again?'

''Scuse me,' said the Elephant's Child, 'but I should not like it at all.'

'How would you like to spank somebody?' said the Bi-Coloured-Python-Rock-Snake.

'I should like it very much indeed,' said the Elephant's Child.

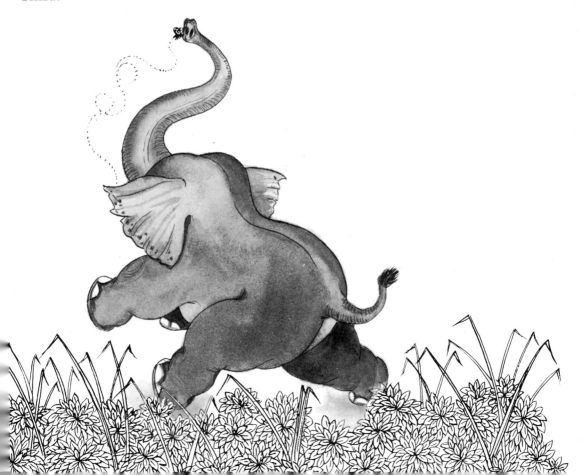

'Well,' said the Bi-Coloured-Python-Rock-Snake, 'you will find that new nose of yours very useful to spank people with.'

'Thank you,' said the Elephant's Child, 'I'll remember that; and now I think I'll go home to all my dear families and try.'

So the Elephant's Child went home across Africa frisking and whisking his trunk. When he wanted fruit to eat he pulled fruit down from a tree, instead of waiting for it to fall as he used to do. When he wanted grass he plucked grass up from the ground, instead of going on his knees as he used to do. When the flies bit him he broke off the branch of a tree and used it as a fly-whisk; and he made himself a new, cool, slushy-squshy mud-cap whenever the sun was hot. When he felt lonely walking through Africa he sang to himself down his trunk, and the noise was louder than several brass bands. He went specially out of his way to find a broad Hippopotamus (she was no relation of his), and he spanked her very hard, to make sure that the Bi-Coloured-Python-Rock-Snake had spoken the truth about his new trunk. The rest of the time he picked up the melon-rinds that he had dropped on his way to the Limpopo – for he was a Tidy Pachyderm.

One dark evening he came back to all his dear families, and he coiled up his trunk and said, 'How do you do?' They were very glad to see him, and immediately said, 'Come here and be spanked for your 'satiable curtiosity.'

'Pooh,' said the Elephant's Child. 'I don't think you peoples know anything about spanking; but I do, and I'll show you.'

Then he uncurled his trunk and knocked two of his dear brothers head over heels.

'O Bananas!' said they, 'where did you learn that trick, and what have you done to your nose?'

'I got a new one from the Crocodile on the banks of the great grey-green, greasy Limpopo River,' said the Elephant's Child. 'I asked him what he had for dinner, and he gave me this to keep.'

'It looks very ugly,' said his hairy uncle, the Baboon.

'It does,' said the Elephant's Child. 'But it's very useful,' and he picked up his hairy uncle, the Baboon, by one hairy leg, and hove him into a hornets' nest.

Then that bad Elephant's Child spanked all his dear families for a long time, till they were very warm and greatly astonished. He pulled out his tall Ostrich aunt's tail-feathers; and he caught his tall uncle, the Giraffe, by the hind-leg, and dragged him through a thorn-bush; and he shouted at his broad aunt, the Hippopotamus, and blew bubbles into her ear when she was sleeping in the water after meals; but he never let any one touch Kolokolo Bird.

At last things grew so exciting that his dear families went off one by one in a hurry to the banks of the great grey-green, greasy Limpopo River, all set about with fever-trees, to borrow new noses from the Crocodile. When they came back nobody spanked anybody any more; and ever since that day, O Best Beloved, all the Elephants you will ever see, besides all those that you won't, have trunks precisely like the trunk of the 'satiable Elephant's Child.

Rudyard Kipling

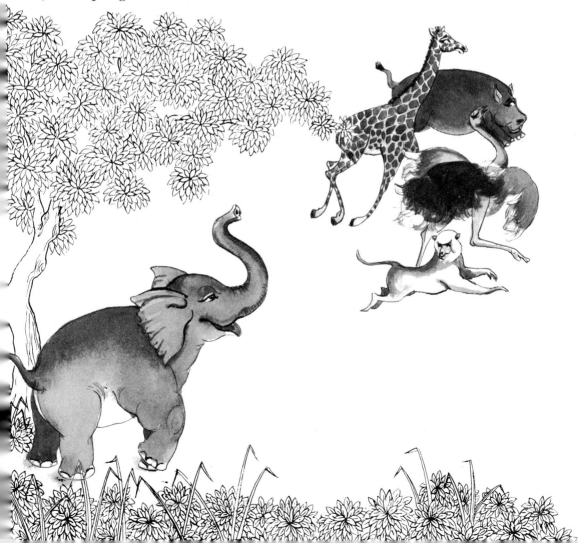

Stuck in the Sand

There was once an elephant who was great friends with a beetle. One day the two friends made up their minds to go for a holiday by the sea.

They reached the sea-shore just as it was getting dark. The elephant picked up driftwood and made a fire. The beetle cooked their tea. Then they stayed up till very late, showing each other how they would swim in the sea.

Next morning the beetle woke up first. He nudged the elephant and together they rushed down to the sea. In went the beetle. He leaped and rolled and dived in the icy water.

But not the elephant.

As soon as he ran into the sea his feet began to sink into the soft, wet sand. Before he had time to think he was stuck fast in the sand. The waves lapped around his tummy.

He yelled to the beetle for help. The beetle tried everything he could think of, but he could not pull his friend out of the sand. While they pulled and tugged and pushed the tide rose slowly. It came higher and higher. The two friends didn't know about tides. They thought the elephant was sinking down further into the sand.

Puffing, the beetle sat on the elephant's head to rest and to think. He saw a fish swim past the elephant's legs.

'Hey, Fish! Stop!' called the beetle. 'My friend is stuck in the sand, and I don't know how to get him out. Can you help?'

The fish looked up at the elephant's tail.

'When I want to move I flick my tail. It never fails.' And the fish swam off, with a flick of his scaly tail.

The beetle and the elephant looked at one another. They both nodded, and the elephant began to flick his little short tail. Nothing happened.

The tide rose a little higher.

'That fish didn't know what he was talking about,' snorted the beetle.

Just then a seagull dived into the water, and bobbed up near the two friends.

'Hey, Seagull! Stop!' yelled the beetle. 'My friend is stuck in the sand, and I don't know how to get him out. Can you help?'

The seagull looked up at the elephant's ears and said, 'When I want to move I flap my wings. It never fails.'

– You don't get down from an elephant. You get down from a duck.

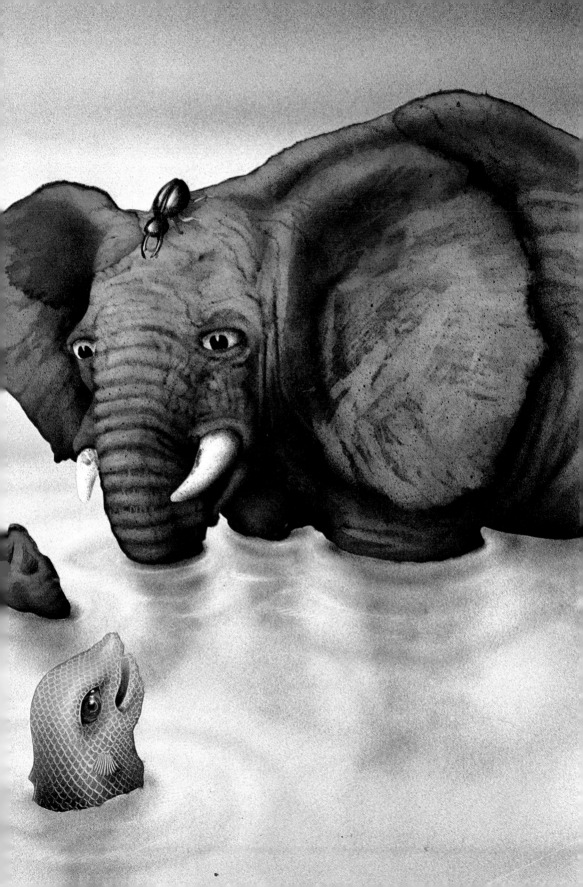

And, with a flap of his wings, he was gone.

The elephant and the beetle looked at one another.

'What a dope,' said the beetle. 'He doesn't mean wings. He must mean your ears.'

'Yes,' agreed the elephant. He began to flap his ears. He flapped and flapped. He flapped until he felt they would drop off. Nothing happened.

But the tide rose a little higher.

There was now more elephant under the water than there was above it.

The beetle was afraid. He sat on his friend's head and thought and thought. As he thought, the tide rose higher and higher. At last a tiny wave washed the beetle right off the elephant's head. At the same moment the elephant floated free of the sand.

'Hooray!' cried the elephant. 'I'm floating. I can swim. How very clever you are, Beetle. You knew it was your weight that was pushing me down into the sand!'

The beetle was very pleased at his friend's words. He was a clever beetle, indeed.

Patricia Adams

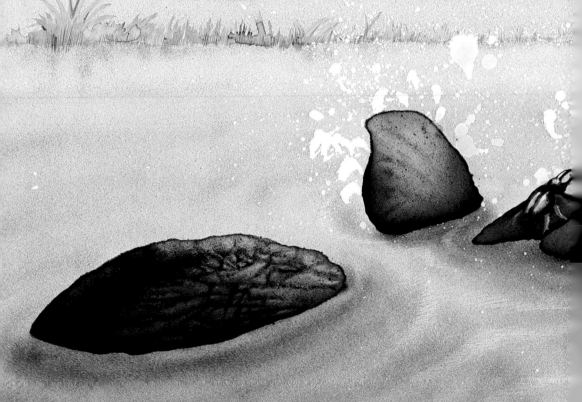

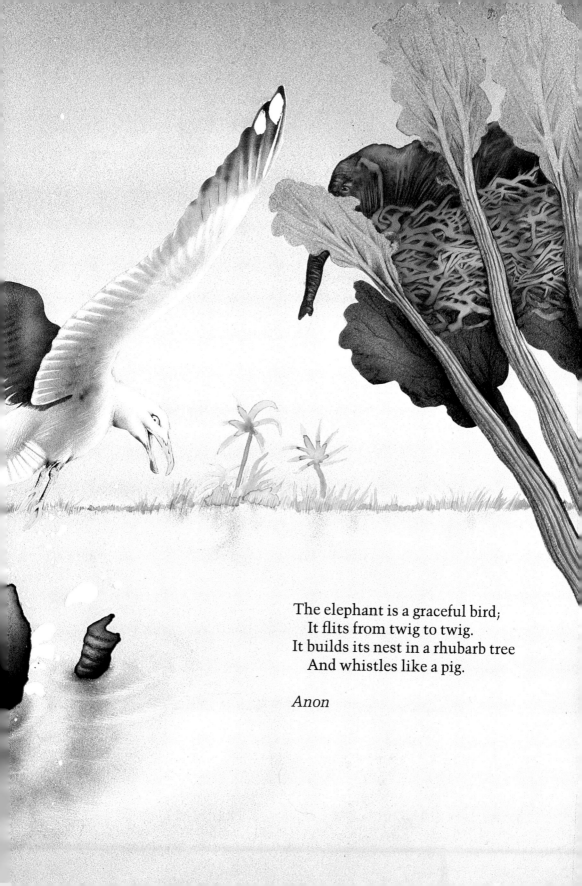

The elephant is a graceful bird;
  It flits from twig to twig.
It builds its nest in a rhubarb tree
  And whistles like a pig.

Anon

A Little Water

Elephant spoke to Rain.

Elephant said: 'If I tore down all the trees and destroyed all growing things, what would you do?'

Rain said: 'If I held back my waters, so that the earth withered and died, what would *you* do?'

And they parted.

Elephant screamed and trumpeted. He tore down all the trees and destroyed all growing things. Silently Rain withheld his waters. The earth withered and died.

There was no water.

Elephant, panting, dug deep into a dried-up water-hole and lay down on his side to keep cool in the fresh soil, but the side of him pressing on the earth withered and died.

Elephant was in agony.

Elephant cried out to Khorhaan: 'You have wings to fly. Take a message to Rain for me. Beg him to give me water.'

Khorhaan went up to Rain, but Rain said: 'No, I will not give him water. He boasted of his strength and power. He tore down all the trees and destroyed all growing things. Let him die.'

Elephant sent Khorhaan a second time: 'Tell him that I have sinned, that I am sorry for my sin. Beg him to listen to me. I pray to him for a little water.'

Rain relented.

First he gave to Khorhaan a white collar to show that he had heard the prayer. Today all Khorhaan's race wear the white collar.

Then Rain's clouds gathered above the dried water-hole where Elephant lay. The clouds lowered and broke, and it was filled with water. Nowhere else did the rain fall.

Elephant rose and drank.

Elephant wanted never to be without water again. He found Tortoise and posted him by the side of the water-hole: 'Guard my water for me. No others may come and drink it.'

And Elephant went to search for food.

Then the panting Lion came, and said: 'The earth burns and I am thirsty. Let me drink.'

Tortoise refused: 'This is Elephant's water. You may not drink.'

The Lion said: 'Stand aside. I will drink.'

Lion drank. All the thirsting animals came to the water and drank.

Elephant returned to find the water-hole dry. 'Tortoise!' he cried. 'Tortoise, where is my water?'

Tortoise said: 'You know I am a small creature. The people take no notice of me. They came and pushed me aside and drank all the water.'

'You shall die,' Elephant said. 'I must consider how. I could crush you beneath my foot.'

'My shell is hard,' said Tortoise. 'If I am to die, I am a thing to be swallowed. Swallow me.'

Elephant swallowed him.

The Tortoise attacked Elephant from within and Elephant was in agony again.

'Tortoise! Good Tortoise!' he cried. 'I was wrong to punish you. Come back and we shall be friends.'

Tortoise took no notice. He bit out Elephant's heart and escaped through a hole in his withered side.

Elephant was dead.

Tortoise was very pleased with himself. 'I will not talk to anyone today, for today I am better than you all,' he boasted. 'Today I got rid of the one you all feared, the one who destroyed the land.'

Kalahari story

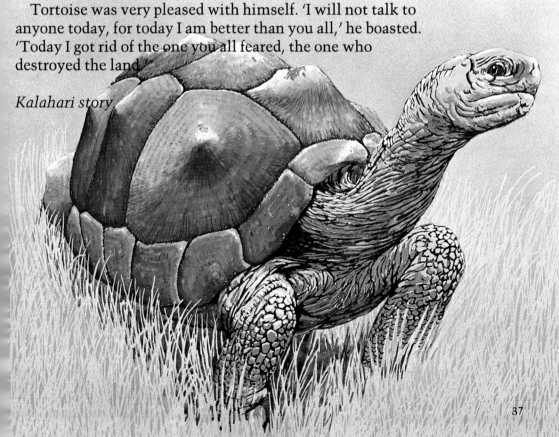

Little Chow Weighs an Elephant

Everyone in the village stared at the elephant. It was the biggest animal they had ever seen. It was two times as tall as a water buffalo. It was fifty times as big as a dog and a hundred times as fat as a goose.

'It *can't* be that big!' everyone said.

But it was.

Tai Tai, Chow Chow, and their son, Little Chow, were looking at the elephant, too.

'Where did it come from?' asked Little Chow. He was eight years old, and he always wanted to know things.

'From far away where the world is hot,' his father said. Chow Chow was the wisest man in the village. He had five long hairs in his eyebrows which showed that he was born wise, and he had two very long fingernails on his left hand, protected by silver fingernail guards. His sleeves were so long they came down over his hands. His long fingernails and long sleeves proved that he did not do any hard work – except study. He knew all the books of Confucius by heart.

Little Chow hoped that some day he would be as wise as his

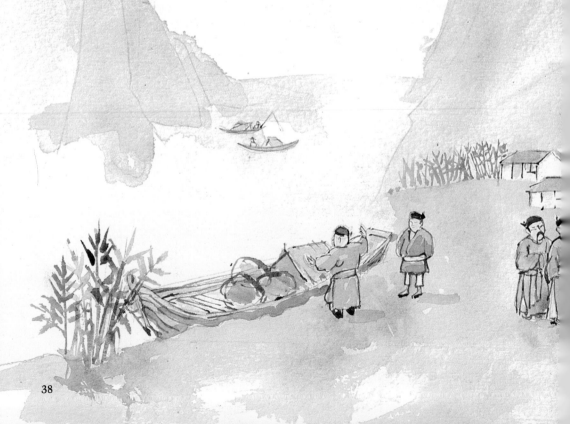

father. 'What does an elephant do?' he asked.

'Who knows?' said his mother. 'It's a gift for the Emperor. He will know what to do with it.'

'How can it go from here to the Emperor?' asked Little Chow. 'The Emperor lives very far away.'

'It will go by barge on the Grand Canal,' Chow Chow replied. 'That is the way everything travels from here to the Emperor.'

The bargeman was looking at the elephant. 'I must know how much it weighs before I take it on my barge,' he said.

'But how can we weigh such a big animal?' asked the people. They scratched their heads and tried to think how to weigh the elephant. No one had scales big enough for the elephant.

Little Chow was thinking and thinking.

'I know how to weigh it,' he said at last. But no one heard him.

'Ask Chow Chow,' the people said. 'He is the wisest man in the village. He will know how to weigh the elephant.'

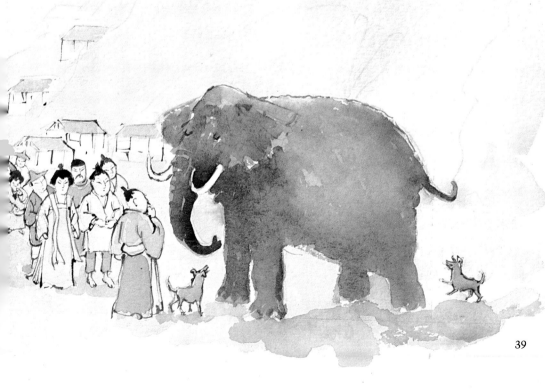

'Bring me a chair,' said Chow Chow. So they brought him a chair. Chow Chow sat down, shut his eyes so that he could think better, and recited all the books of Confucius – from beginning to end. Then he opened his eyes and said, 'Confucius does not say how to weigh an elephant.'

'Ai! Ai!' the people said. 'What shall we do now?'

'I know how to weigh it,' Little Chow said again, a little louder this time.

'Be quiet,' whispered his mother. 'Let wise people talk.'

Then everyone thought some more.

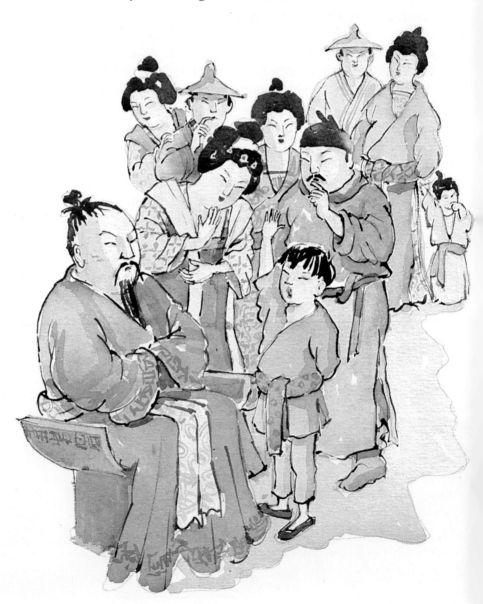

'Weigh one leg at a time,' said one.

'Put the elephant on a lot of scales and add up the weight,' said another.

'I know how to do it,' insisted Little Chow. But nobody listened.

'Don't weigh it at all,' said Tai Tai. 'Just put it on the barge and send it to the Emperor.'

All the people nodded their heads. 'Yes, that is the best thing to do. If the Emperor wants to know how much the elephant weighs, he will find a way to weigh it.'

'Quite right,' said Tai Tai. 'Who cares how much it weighs?'

'I care,' the bargeman said. 'I charge by weight. I must know how much the elephant weighs.'

'You should do it free for the Emperor,' said Tai Tai, and all the people agreed.

'"Free for the Emperor" is all right for rich people,' said the bargeman, 'but "free for the Emperor" will not feed me nor my father and mother, nor my wife and four sons and three daughters, nor my brothers who help me on the barge, nor their families. To say nothing of my water buffalo.'

Everyone nodded. They knew the bargeman was right.

'Who is sending this gift to the Emperor?' asked Tai Tai.

'Mr Lee, of course. No one else is rich enough to send an elephant to the Emperor.'

'Then let Mr Lee pay you something, bargeman, and take the elephant without weighing it.'

'That is not the proper way to do things,' said the bargeman stubbornly. 'The elephant must be weighed.'

'There is no way for us to to weigh an elephant,' said the people, shaking their heads.

Then Little Chow pushed his way to the front and said very loudly, '*I know how to weigh the elephant!*'

This time everyone heard him, and everyone laughed. The men laughed, the women laughed, and all the boys and girls laughed and pointed their fingers at Little Chow.

'But I *do* know how!' Little Chow said.

'Ai! Ai!' said Chow Chow. 'My son has lost his senses.'

'Ai! Ai!' said Tai Tai. 'He is making my face red.'

'Well, let's hear it,' the people said. 'If you are so wise, Little Chow, tell us how to weigh this elephant.' But they laughed when they said it.

Little Chow didn't mind. 'Put the elephant on the barge,' he said.

'The elephant has not been weighed yet,' protested the bargeman.

'This is how to weigh it,' said Little Chow. 'Put the elephant on the barge.'

'The barge isn't a scale, you know,' the people said.

'I know,' Little Chow replied patiently. 'I will tell you how to weigh the elephant. First put it on the barge.'

So the people led the elephant on to the barge.

'Now what?' they asked.

'Now,' said little Chow, 'do you see where the water comes up to on the side of the barge? Make a mark there, all around.'

'Well!' said the people. 'This is a strange way to weigh an elephant.' But they marked the side of the barge next to the land, and then the bargeman turned the barge around and they marked the other side.

'Now take the elephant off,' Little Chow said.

'Then what was all that work for, marking the barge?' the people muttered.

'Wait and see,' said Little Chow.

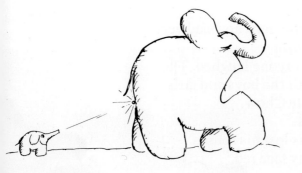
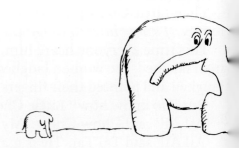

So the people led the elephant off again and gave it some leaves to eat because it was getting cross.

Then everyone looked at Little Chow to see what he would say next.

Little Chow smiled and took a deep breath. 'Now,' he said, 'fill the barge with stones until the water comes up to the mark you made, and then take the stones off and weigh them a few at a time. Add it all up and you will know how much the elephant weighs.'

'Aiyah!'' everyone said.

'Of course!'

'Why didn't we think of that?'

'*That* is how to weigh an elephant!'

And then they all said, 'What a wise boy! When he grows up he will be almost as wise as his father!'

Chow Chow put his hand on Little Chow's shoulder. 'Wiser, I think,' he said.

'Of course,' said Tai Tai. 'He is my son.'

So the people weighed the elephant just as Little Chow had told them to, and the bargeman took it to the Emperor.

Jean Kennedy

– You would hear a loud screaming noise.

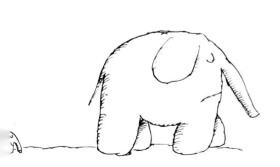
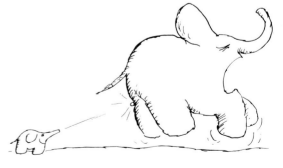

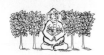

Only One Fleece

Once an elephant was appointed king of the forest. It is well known that elephants are very intelligent, but it happened that this one was a bit of a fool. Not wicked, you understand, but foolish.

One day the sheep came to him with a petition. The wolves were tearing them to pieces and would the king please make them stop.

'Oh, you rogues!' cried the elephant. 'How dare you do this! It must stop at once.'

'Your Majesty,' said the wolves, 'you should not believe everything the sheep tell you. Allow us to explain before you give judgment.'

'I'm listening,' said the elephant.

'Your Majesty knows that sheep are covered in wool. Indeed, they have so much they can hardly run for it. Your Majesty has already given permission for us to take wool from the sheep so that we shall not go cold in winter. That's all we've done. They complain because they're just stupid sheep. We take a single fleece from each sheep we meet and they grumble even about that. One little fleece is not very much.'

'One fleece?' asked the elephant.

'One,' said the wolves.

'That can't be so bad. All right, then. One fleece and no more. I shall not tolerate any injustice. If you take more than a single fleece from each sheep I shall punish you.'

'Of course, Your Majesty,' said the wolves, and smiled.

Ivan Krylov

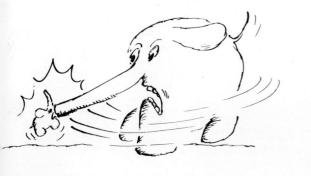

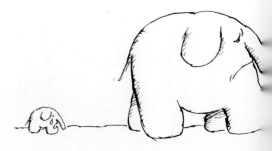

Oliphaunt

Grey as a mouse,
Big as a house,
Nose like a snake,
I make the earth shake,
As I tramp through the grass;
Trees crack as I pass.
With horns in my mouth
I walk in the South,
Flapping big ears.
Beyond count of years
I stump round and round,
Never lie on the ground,
Not even to die.
Oliphaunt am I,
Biggest of all,
Huge, old, and tall.
If ever you'd met me,
You wouldn't forget me.
If you never do,
You won't think I'm true;
But old Oliphaunt am I,
And I never lie.

J. R. R. Tolkien

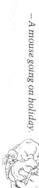

– *A mouse going on holiday.*

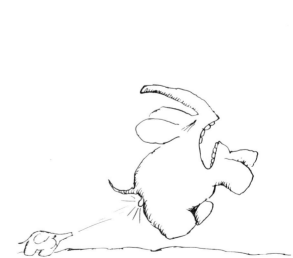

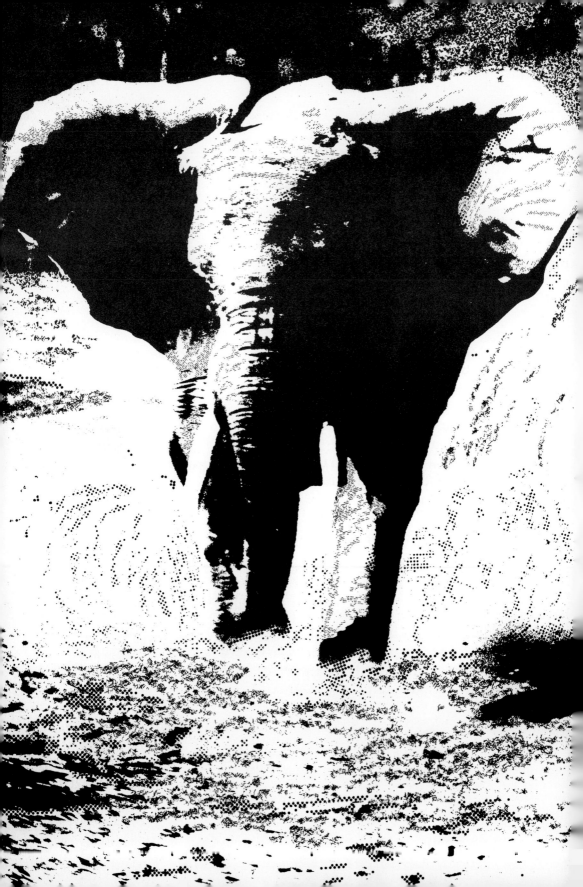

Attacked by an Elephant

In July 1959, an African roads superintendent was cycling through Murchison Falls Park to the hospital at Masindi because his pregnant wife had been taken ill there. In his haste, he suddenly found himself in the middle of a herd of elephants some miles down the road.

'There were elephants to the left of me, to the right of me, in front of me and behind me – elephants everywhere. I got off my bicycle and stood there for a while without moving. My presence didn't seem to have startled them, although they eyed me closely. After a short time the animals began to move off and my fear subsided. Then, suddenly, one mother-elephant attacked me from the flank and another from the front. I threw down my bicycle and ran faster than I had ever run before.

'The she-elephant took no notice of the bicycle, so I threw her my big overcoat. That didn't interest her either, so I jettisoned a shoe. She didn't want the shoe, so I picked up a stick. The elephant grabbed the other end of the stick, and we continued to run like that. I felt as if I was flying, but I tired very quickly. I lost ground whereas the elephant ran faster and faster. Just as I felt her trunk almost touching me I tripped and fell between her forelegs. The cow lowered her massive head and gored the ground with her tusks, pinning me between them.

'I somehow managed, in my desperation, to slip out of my jacket and thrust it right into the mouth of the furious beast with my left hand. She kicked me with her foot and ran off. I lay there on the ground, half stunned, but managed to crawl another two hundred yards or so on my knees. When I had fully recovered consciousness I went back to the road-workers' camp. From there someone took me by bicycle to Masindi Hospital, where I received treatment.'

Bernhard Grzimek

How to become Popular

Once, when the lion was king, it so happened that the
elephant was very popular among the lions.

'How has he managed it?' the other animals asked. 'No one
could say he's beautiful, he isn't bright and he's not even
funny. He has bad manners and bad habits. Very bad habits.'
And they continued to talk about all the elephant's faults.

The fox waved her tail. 'I could understand it,' she said, 'if
he had a fine bushy tail like mine.'

'Or, sister,' said the bear, 'if he had a good set of claws.
Then I wouldn't have been a bit surprised. But we all know he
hasn't got any claws at all.'

'Perhaps it's his tusks,' the ox said. 'It's just possible
they've mistaken them for horns.'

The ass shook his ears. 'You really don't know?' he said.
'Why, I can tell you. He would never have got where he is if
he hadn't had such fine, big ears.'

Ivan Krylov

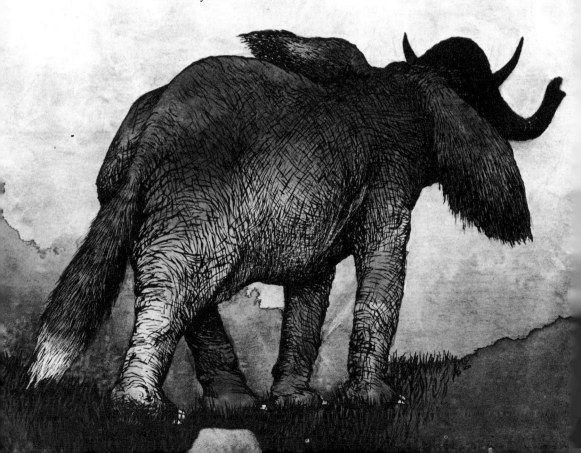

How Anansi got his Shape

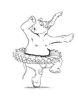

Once Elephant owned a very fine cow. He boasted that it was the finest cow in the Bush and called all the other animals to come and admire it.

'And what's more,' he said, 'I will give this cow to any of you if you'll let me give you a blow as well. Just one blow.' Elephant was proud of his strength.

No one accepted – no one, that is, until Anansi heard about it. He was, as usual, very hungry.

'O Lord of the Bush,' he said. 'I will take your cow and a blow from you.'

So Elephant gave Anansi the cow. 'Take the cow now,' he said. 'On Friday I shall come and give you the blow I owe you.'

Anansi took the cow home and killed it. He and his family were not hungry any more, but when Friday came Anansi was very frightened. He didn't know what to do. In the end he worked out a plan with his wife. She took the groundnuts out of a shell and put Anansi in instead, covering the hole up. She then threw him out into the corner of the yard where one of their fowls immediately gobbled him up, shell and all.

Elephant came. 'Where is Anansi?' he said. 'I have something for him.'

'He has gone to the farm.'

Elephant refused to believe her and got very angry.

'Fetch me the bakologo man!' he cried.

Bakologo man soon came. Elephant explained what had happened and told him that now he wanted to know where Anansi was hiding. Bakologo consulted his magic. Soon he said. 'Anansi is inside a groundnut shell inside the fowl.'

Elephant killed the bird, found the groundnut, broke it open and took out Anansi. 'Why do you hide from me?'

Anansi knew one blow from Elephant would kill him and begged for his life.

'We were hungry,' he said. 'We needed food to stay alive.' Indeed, Anansi had hoped to find a way of avoiding Elephant until he had forgotten about the matter. 'O Lord,' he added, 'you do not need to hit me for me to know how strong you are.'

In the end Elephant was sorry for Anansi. 'That is true,' he said, 'but still you have taken my cow. Instead of one hard blow I shall give you twelve small taps, the first now, the second next Friday and so on.'

And he gave Anansi his first tap.

Now a tap from an elephant is no laughing matter. This one drove Anansi's head down into his shoulders so that even today he has no neck.

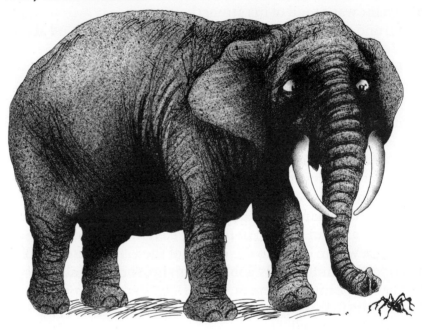

When Friday drew near Anansi was in a great fix. He had no new ideas, so he decided to risk the groundnut trick again. 'And when Elephant comes,' he said to his wife, 'you must tell him I've gone right away from here.'

He got inside a groundnut shell and told his wife to throw him well away from the house this time. She sealed the shell, took it outside and threw it into the Bush. Again one of the fowls found him and ate him up.

That night a wild cat found the fowl, caught her and ate her.

In the morning a dog saw the cat, caught her and ate her.

Later a hyena came across the dog, caught him and ate him.

Then a lion stalked the hyena, caught her and ate her.

The lion went down to the water for a drink. As he stretched over the water a python caught hold of him and swallowed him.

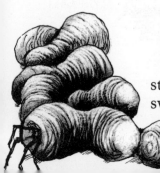

'Where is Anansi?' Elephant demanded when he arrived on Friday morning.

'Oh, he's gone away, right away. He didn't say where. He didn't say when he would be back.'

'Fetch the bakologo man!' Elephant was really angry this time.

Bakologo man bent over his magic and muttered to himself. 'Come with me,' he said at last, and took Elephant down to the riverside. He showed Elephant the sleeping python and told him to kill it.

Elephant killed the python and found the lion.

He cut open the lion and found the hyena.

He cut open the hyena and found the dog.

He cut open the dog and found the cat.

He cut open the cat and found the fowl.

He cut open the fowl and found the groundnut.

And inside the groundnut he found Anansi.

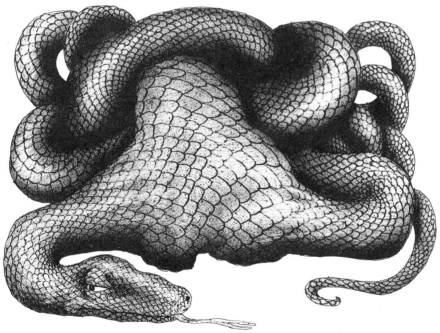

'Do you think that I, Lord of all the Bush, should chase after a bakologo man because of you? Do you think I should spend time over a miserable little thing that can't keep a bargain and won't take his punishment? This time you will really get the blow I promised you. What do you say?'

And Anansi could only·beg for his life.

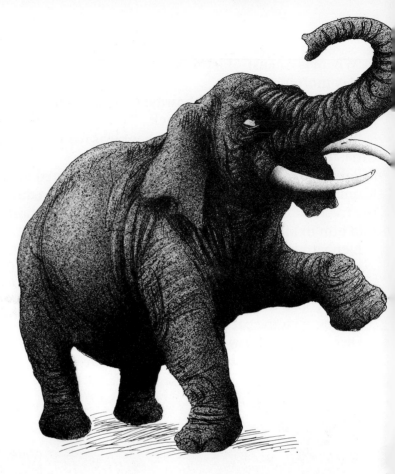

Elephant would not listen, and frightened Anansi begged harder and harder.

'Have you friends?' said Elephant at last. 'Who will come and speak for you?'

Anansi could think only of Bambua, the little Red Duiker, but when he came he said, 'No, I will not beg for you. You brought this trouble on yourself and you deserve Elephant's punishment for it. Besides, when you got your food did you think of my hunger? You offered me none of it.'

By now Elephant's anger had cooled a little, and he began to feel sorry for the frightened little creature in front of him.

'All right,' he said, 'it is over. You are too wretched for me to bother about. Get out!' And he gave Anansi a kick.

Now a kick from an elephant is no laughing matter and Anansi was hurled against a tree. That is why today, as well as having no neck, Anansi is quite flat. In those days he was much fatter.

Dagomba story

The Match

One empty afternoon, when there was nothing at all to do, the elephants and the mice decided to have a game of football. They were soon hard at it and other animals gathered round to watch.

It was clear the elephants were no match for the mice, who were leading 5–0 at half time. Changing ends made no difference. Then, just as one brilliant little mouse was about to shoot for goal – it would have been his hat trick – the opposing centre-half trod on him. There was a very nasty scene and the match was abandoned as the spectators streamed on to the pitch. Some had to hold the mice back to stop them from attacking the elephants; others surrounded the guilty elephant who was being told off by the referee.

'I'm sorry!' he kept saying. 'I didn't mean it. I didn't mean it. I just tried to trip him!'

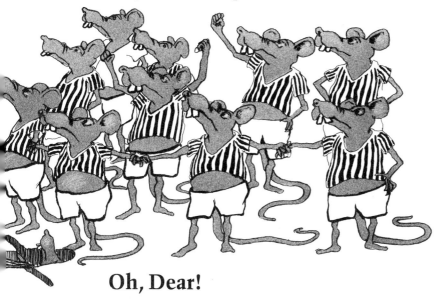

Oh, Dear!

Once there was an elephant who didn't look where she was going and trod on a hen. She was very upset, especially when she looked down and saw all the chicks running about cheeping.

'Oh, dear!' she said. 'Poor little things! I'd better look after them now.'

So, remembering how mother hens behave, she tenderly gathered all the chicks together and sat on them.

The Elephant on Daddy's Car

'Mummy,' said Jeremy James, 'there's an elephant sitting on Daddy's car.'

'Yes, dear,' said Mummy, eyes fixed on hands fixed on dough fixed on table.

'Mummy, why is the elephant sitting on Daddy's car?'

'I expect it's tired, dear. It'll probably get up and go away soon.'

'Well, it hasn't,' said Jeremy James two minutes later. 'It hasn't got up. The car's gone down, but the elephant hasn't got up. Mummy, do you think I ought to tell Daddy?'

'No, no, leave your father,' said Mummy, 'you know he hates being interrupted when he's working.'

'Daddy's watching a football match on television.'

'If Daddy says he's working, he's working.'

'Well, there's an elephant sitting on his car,' said Jeremy James.

Mummy thumbed sultanas into the dough to make eyes and noses.

'And the car doesn't look very happy about it,' said Jeremy James.

'Jeremy James,' said Mummy. 'Elephants don't sit on cars.'

'Well this one does.'

'Elephants don't sit on cars. If Mummy says elephants don't sit on cars, dear, then elephants don't sit on cars.'

'But . . .'

'They don't. Finish! Now play with your train set.'

Jeremy James sat on the carpet, and played with his train set, and thought about the elephant on Daddy's car, and thought about how stubborn Mummies can be when they want to be, and how if he was a Mummy and his son said there was an elephant on Daddy's car, he would say 'What a clever boy,' and 'Thank you for telling me,' and 'Here's some money for an ice-cream.' Instead of just 'Elephants don't sit on cars.'

'Goal!' said the television set in the sitting-room.

'Goal!' said Daddy, hard at work.

And the elephant was still sitting on Daddy's car.

'Mummy,' said Jeremy James, for the latest development really couldn't be ignored. 'Mummy, the elephant has just

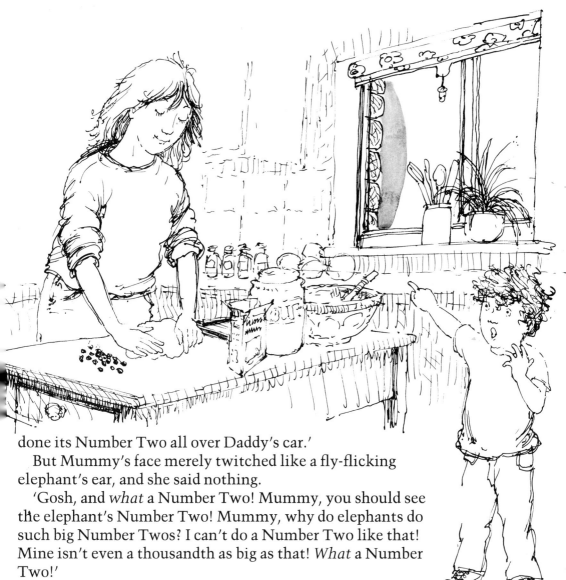

done its Number Two all over Daddy's car.'

But Mummy's face merely twitched like a fly-flicking elephant's ear, and she said nothing.

'Gosh, and *what* a Number Two! Mummy, you should see the elephant's Number Two! Mummy, why do elephants do such big Number Twos? I can't do a Number Two like that! Mine isn't even a thousandth as big as that! *What* a Number Two!'

'Jeremy James, if you go on talking like that, I shall send you straight to bed. Now play with your train set, and let's have no more elephant talk, and certainly no more about Number Twos. Do you hear?'

'Yes, Mummy.'

No Number Twos. Anyone would think that Number Twos were unhealthy. Only look what happened when you didn't do a Number Two. Then it was: 'Jeremy James, have you done your Number Two? You haven't done your Number Two? Then sit there until you have.' Now tell them an elephant's done his Number Two on Daddy's car, and suddenly it's rude. Why can't grown-ups make up their minds?

Jeremy James played with his train set.

Jeremy James looked out of the window. The elephant was gone.

'Mummy,' said Jeremy James.

'What is it now?' said Mummy, half in and half out of the oven.

'The elephant's gone.'

'Hmmph.'

That was a typical grown-up word: 'Hmmph.' It was for grown-ups only, and meant whatever they wanted it to mean. Jeremy James had tried to use a 'Hmmph' once himself. Mummy had said, 'Have you done your Number Two?' (at one of those times when Number Two wasn't rude) and he'd replied 'Hmmph', because that was how grown-ups got out of awkward questions like Will you buy me something nice today, or Why can't I have a toy racing car like Timothy's? Only Jeremy James obviously didn't know how to use it, because Mummy told him to speak properly, even though he'd said 'Hmmph' perfectly properly.

Daddy came out of the sitting-room, with his face as long as an elephant's nose.

'They lost,' said Daddy. 'Right at the end. An own goal.'

Then Daddy leaned on the kitchen doorpost as he always did when he'd been working (and sometimes when he *was* working), and watched Mummy working, presumably to make sure she was doing everything right. Jeremy James had tried leaning on the doorpost once and saying, as Daddy always ended up by saying, 'Will it be long, dear?' But instead of getting Mummy's normal 'Hmmph', he'd had a 'Now don't you start!' and been sent off to play with his train set, which he was sick of anyway.

'Will it be long, dear?' said Daddy.

'Hmmph,' said Mummy.

'Now don't you start,' said Jeremy James quietly.

'An own goal,' said Daddy. 'Right at the end.'

'Was that goal Number Two?' asked Jeremy James.

'I don't know what's got into that child,' said Mummy.

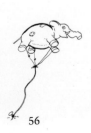

Daddy elbowed himself upright off the doorpost, took one hand out of one pocket ('Take your hands out of your pockets, Jeremy James!'), yawned, and announced, 'Maybe I'll go and clean the car.'

Mummy didn't say, 'There won't be time before tea,' though Daddy waited quite a long time for her to say it, and so Daddy eventually left the kitchen, crossed the dining-room, entered the hall, opened the front door, and went out of the house.

Jeremy James stood at the window and wondered what new words Daddy would use.

Daddy didn't use any words. Daddy's mouth fell open, and then Daddy came back to the house, opened the front door, entered the hall, crossed the dining-room, and held himself up by the kitchen doorpost.

'The car!' said Daddy. Then his mouth opened and shut several times as if he'd just been pulled out of the water. 'The car!' he said again.

'What's the matter with it?' asked Mummy, spreading hand-cream over the bread.

'It's ruined! It ... it ... it's ruined! It looks as if it's been completely squashed! Completely and utterly squashed!'

'Oh John,' said Mummy, who only called Daddy John when she was very upset or when she wanted some money, 'Oh John, there ... there isn't ... um ... sort of ... dung all over it as well, is there?'

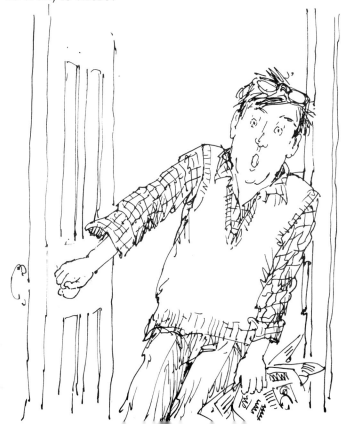

'Yes,' said Daddy, 'there jolly well is! I've never seen anything like it, either. Must have been a herd of cows dancing on the thing!'

'It wasn't a herd of cows,' said Jeremy James, 'it was an elephant. And I saw it. And I told Mummy, but she wouldn't listen.'

'An elephant!' said Daddy. 'You saw an elephant on the car?'

'Yes,' said Jeremy James, 'and I saw it do its Number Two as well.'

'Then why the . . . . didn't one of you tell me?'

'Hmmph!' said Mummy, and Jeremy James played with his train set.

David Henry Wilson

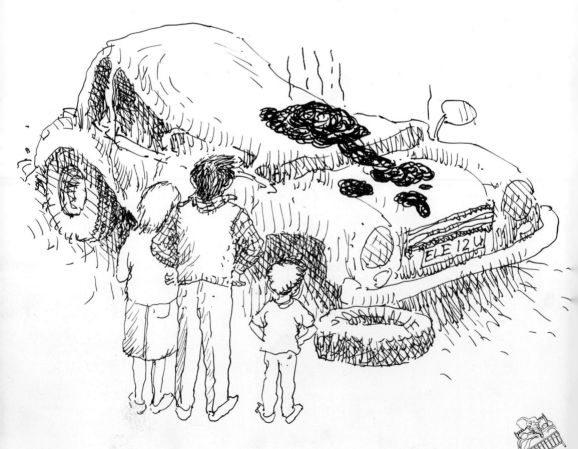

– You can smell the peanuts on his breath.

Elephants are different to different people

Wilson and Pilcer and Snack stood before the zoo elephant.

Wilson said, 'What is its name? Is it from Asia or Africa?
Who feeds it? Is it a he or a she? How old is it? Do they have
twins? How much does it cost to feed? How much does it
weigh? If it dies, how much will another one cost? If it dies,
what will they use the bones, the fat, and the hide for? What
use is it besides to look at?'

Pilcer didn't have any questions; he was murmuring to
himself, 'It's a house by itself, walls and windows, the ears
came from tall cornfields, by God; the architect of those legs
was a workman, by God; he stands like a bridge out across
deep water, the face is sad and the eyes are kind, I know
elephants are good to babies.'

Snack looked up and down and at last said to himself, 'He's
a tough son-of-a-gun outside and I'll bet he's got a strong
heart, I'll bet he's strong as a copper-riveted boiler inside.'

They didn't put up any arguments.
They didn't throw anything in each other's faces.
Three men saw the elephant three ways
And let it go at that.
They didn't spoil a sunny Sunday afternoon;
'Sunday comes only once a week,' they told each other.

Carl Sandburg

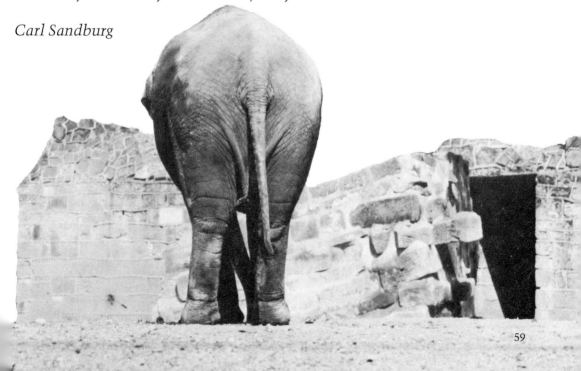

The End of a Land-Rover

Only the elephants' backs were visible above the bush as my stripped-down Land-Rover edged towards them. Mary, the other large old cow in this family, standing in a small clearing, barely looked up from her food, but she shook her head in mild irritation when a thicket splintered as I drove over it. I was glad to see them as they had been missing for over a month.

Mhoja, standing in the back, spotted another group, composed of strangers, which he could see through the foliage. I drove towards them, crushing branches in the way. In front of me a young female with a small calf whom I could not recognize, ran off in alarm, behind a gardenia bush. Seconds later a huge, bow-tusked female came headlong round the gardenia and without uttering a sound, nor pausing in her stride, plunged her tusks up to the gums into the body of my Land-Rover. Mhoja, and a temporary labourer Simeon, who had remained standing in the back just behind the cab, saw the tusks appear beneath their feet and with the huge shape looming over them, jumped out of the car and vanished into the bush.

The first shock threw the car half round. The elephant pulled her tusks out and thrust them in again.

'Don't get out of the car,' I shouted to Katie. She lay down on the floor.

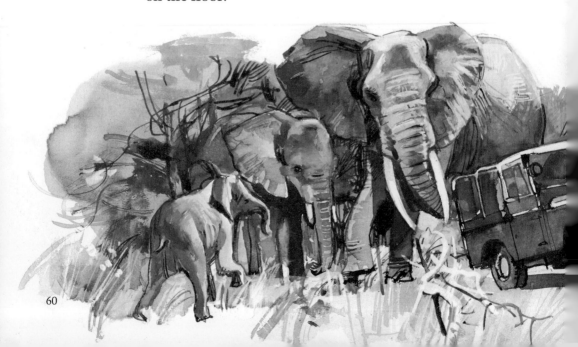

Now more elephants with babies in the forefront burst out of the bush on the right and joined in the attack. A three-year-old calf butted the mudguard and then stood back bewildered. Fortunately, because of our relative sizes, only three elephants could concentrate on the Land-Rover at one time, but it was enough. It felt half-way between being a rugger ball in a scrum, and a dinghy overtaken by three contradictory tidal waves. The car teetered on the point of balance but just missed overturning. Tusks were thrust in and withdrawn with great vigour. Loud and continuous trumpeting rent the air, together with that fatal sound of tearing metal. However, I was not thinking just then about my new Land-Rover, because an enormous brown eye embedded in gnarled skin with long eyelashes materialized through the upper door. This belonged to a cow who was using the weight of her head to force down the roof of the cab. The cab cracked and gave, but then held firm, while her tusks ripped sideways across the door. I could have touched the eye with my fingers. To my relief it disappeared without apparently perceiving that it had been looking at the undamaged brain of this metal animal. I could imagine her picking off our heads just like bananas off a bunch.

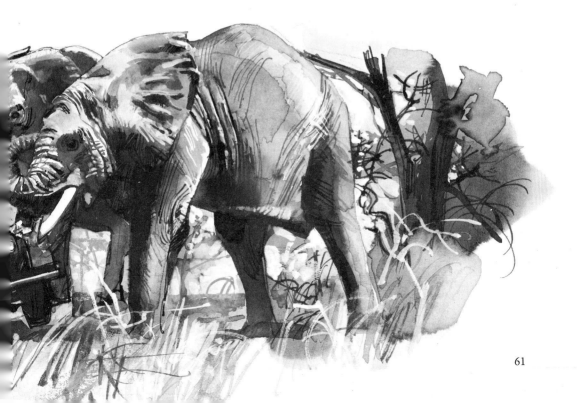

A huge latecomer with as much zeal as the rest put together now came into contact with the front. One wing folded up like paper and a tusk went through the radiator. She stabbed again and wrenched her embedded tusks upwards like a demented fork lift. Then digging her tusks in again she charged, and the Land-Rover was carried backwards at high speed for thirty-five yards until it squashed up against an ant heap surmounted by a small tree.

They left us now at rest, adorning the ant heap, and retired thirty yards where they formed a tight circle and after a few excited trumpets and growls, dissolved into the bush, with streaks of green paint on their tusks.

Iain Douglas-Hamilton

Tromp! Tromp!

The elephant has such BIG FEET,
He really is a wonder!
    Through the jungle, up and down,
    The animals for miles around
      Hear the TROMP-TROMP elephant sound
And think it must be thunder!
      TROMP!
      TROMP!
      TROMP!

Kathryn Taylor

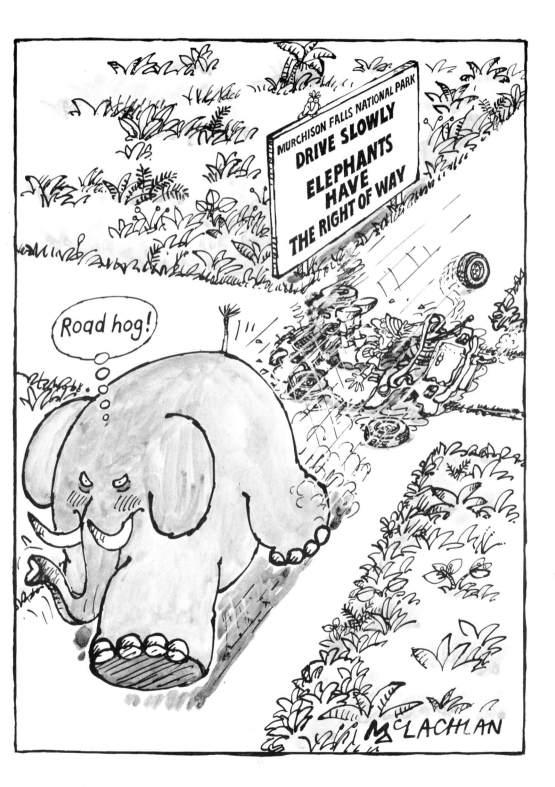

The Force of Habit

A tail behind, a trunk in front,
Complete the usual elephant.
The tail in front, the trunk behind,
Is what you very seldom find.
If you for specimens should hunt
With trunks behind and tails in front.
That hunt would occupy you long;
The force of habit is so strong.

A. E. Housman

When people call this beast to mi
They marvel more and more
At such a *little* tail behind,
So LARGE a trunk before.

Hilaire Belloc

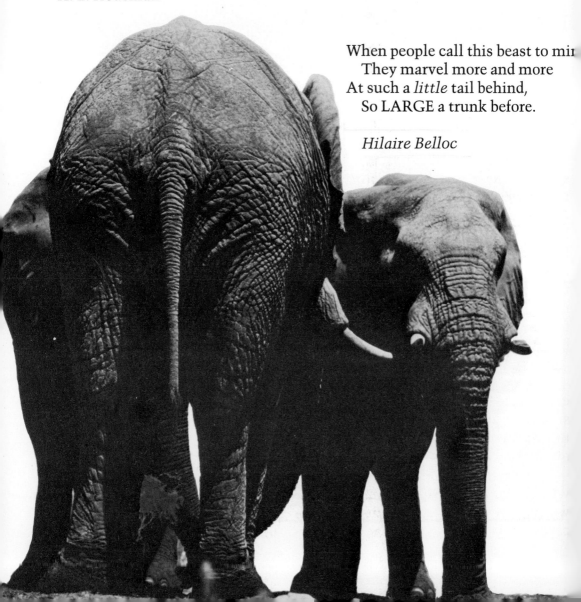

N'Dombo

The two old elephants came to a halt. Young N'Dombo, who had led the way through the dense forest, stopped too. The two old bulls found the sudden burst of bright blue daylight dazzling after the steaming green glow of the forest.

To them it was an unknown land and they were scared, for suddenly the sky was no longer supported by tree-tops; it was too high, too wide. And the sun made everything glitter and hurt their eyes.

The old ones had come with N'Dombo as far as this but they refused to go any farther. N'Dombo had brought them all the way from the mountains, trekking on, day and night, without stopping.

He stretched his trunk now beyond this green world of theirs to where the valley appeared. They knew very well that their way was through that valley where man's bush began. They twisted and extended their trunks to take in the various smells that rose from the villages dotted here and there upon the distant plain.

Was it possible that out of all these unknown mingling scents N'Dombo would be able to tell the one he was looking for? No, he would never find it. The two old bulls trampled the ground, grumbling. They realized now that the whole idea had been mad from the start. They remembered what N'Dombo had told them of his life among men – marvellous but terrifying memories. When the elders of the elephant tribe had held their grand council round their chief, who lay mortally wounded, they never should have let N'Dombo talk, for he had been bewitched by his experience of man's bushland.

No, they would go no farther.

But nothing could deter N'Dombo now; he felt so deeply excited to be back. Even at the edge of the forest these things spoke to him with the voice of man – and what an unforgettable voice that was! Once you had heard it, it went on ringing in your ears long afterwards.

No wonder the elders of the tribe could never understand why N'Dombo was different from the rest! The fact was, he would never be just an animal any more. For he had been captured in the great bush when he was still a little calf not

yet weaned and he had been suckled on cows' milk and had
spent a great part of his young life with men.

The two old ones watched N'Dombo go striding away.
Presently they gave up trying to follow his scent, for it was
being wafted away by the wind. He was lost to them in the
land of man.

They turned away and started back along the shady
corridors of the green kingdom through which they had come,
and the forest closed behind them. When they reached the
tribe again they would tell them how N'Dombo had gone on
alone, to meet the fearsome creature which goes on two feet;
he had gone on alone to find the village called Tenga which he
remembered.

N'Dombo kept on without a stop for the whole of one long
day. In the evening he came to the river and then he only had
to follow its thread of blue water. It ran through the grass,
threading its way between rocks and then spreading out into a
large pool where the water rested, clear and smooth.

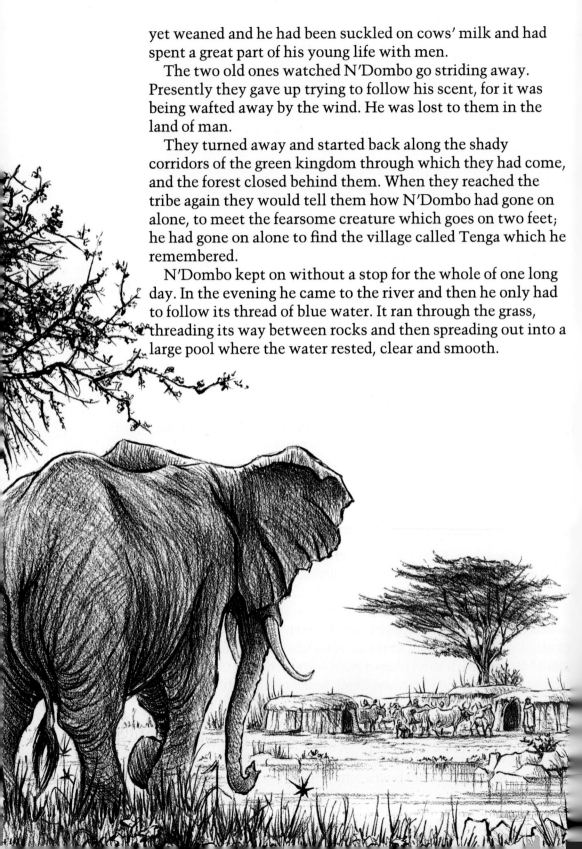

N'Dombo knew this pool. He knew the hill that rose before him. He recognized all the features of this little universe. It was here that he had spent his early days when he was a calf. To think that then he had drunk the milk of these tiny creatures. This evening, as he gazed at the cows, they seemed to him minute.

And how small the village was! The huts looked squashed. These animals hopping about outside them like fleas, jumping and bouncing about with hoarse shouts, were the house dogs. N'Dombo had recognized them. Yes, they must be dogs, these flying fleas!

'It's me – N'Dombo!'

But of course it was no good expecting fleas to listen. They were just throwing the whole village into an uproar. Women came out of their huts and fled in panic, yelling:

'N'Dombo! N'Dombo!'

And yet they knew his name! 'N'Dombo – elephant,' they shouted, and ran away!

So N'Dombo stayed there swaying from one foot to the other, feeling enormous and clumsy and not daring to step any farther for fear of crushing one of these little huts.

'It's me – N'Dombo!' He did all he could to tone down his brassy voice.

At last came a reply, the sad, gentle lowing of an old red cow with horns that curved right round on her forehead. His old humped nurse had recognized him and stretched out her nose towards him. She craned her thin neck to try and see this monstrous baby of hers whose head was up in the sky.

N'Dombo hardly heard the noise of the panic-stricken village now. The men were coming out brandishing their bows, spears, and lances, but he did not hear their shouts, nor the shrill call of their hunting whistles and the iron clatter and rattle of arms. Everything had become so small. There was only one thing still the right size for the elephants and that was the tree. Even in its young days it was huge; its shade spread over all the homes of these men and their humped cattle. It was here, at the foot of the tree, that Wanga, the chief's son, used to tie up the red cow and then fetch his pet elephant calf to be fed.

How frightened that poor cow had been at first! How she used to tug on the rope all the time Wanga was talking to her!

She used to calm down a little when N'Dombo started flicking the flies off her with a branch he tore from the tree. Then he would suck greedily and she stood patiently still, tired with fright.

But she had soon grown used to him. N'Dombo remembered everything. Those early days came back to him with a feeling of great joy.

His nurse must be waiting for him to pluck a big leafy branch now as he used to do and stroke her flanks. He reached up his trunk into the tree, found the thickest branch near the top, and snapped it off. Then with this gigantic bough he stroked his nurse's old red hide.

Now the men came running up wanting to play, just like the band of wild boys Wanga had led in the past. N'Dombo had forgotten nothing. He remembered all those games Wanga had taught him and he felt sure he could still play the animal's part.

Their best game was a sort of hunt, led by Wanga, with N'Dombo for the prey. N'Dombo used to hide, then Wanga and his boys would crawl through the grass, stalking him, ambush him with a shower of little arrows, and rush out waving sharpened sticks for lances. At this point N'Dombo was supposed to charge, but he had found it difficult to understand that he was expected to attack his friends.

But Wanga was fearless. He used to fly into a rage when N'Dombo stepped back instead of taking the offensive; for N'Dombo did not want to throw his whole weight upon the small hunters for fear of hurting them. So Wanga had taught him the wild elephants' rules of warfare and all the dodges they resorted to when chased.

N'Dombo remembered it all . . . He used to swish his trunk from side to side without breaking any legs, while the boys tore about wildly excited and finally surrounded him for the best part of all: the capture. They chased him to where they had strung a tangle of creepers between the trees. N'Dombo went into it full tilt and got his legs caught, stumbled and rolled over like a ball, and the boys threw themselves upon him yelling and climbed all over him.

The game ended with Wanga's triumphal march home perched on his fettered prize – for another thing his young master had trained N'Dombo to do was to pick him up in his trunk, lift him, and put him on his neck.

On this memorable evening of N'Dombo's return, with all this hullabaloo, all the men of the village seemed to want to join in the game and celebrate his return. Real arrows and spears flew in all directions – and N'Dombo, thrilled and excited, trumpeted his war-cry and threw himself whole-heartedly into this extraordinary hunt-game. He did not feel the sharp arrows pierce his hide and his ears. He did not see his blood dripping from the spears he pulled out with his trunk. Their iron points ripped his skin and many javelins remained in his flesh because he could not reach them.

But where was Wanga all this time? What was he doing?
'N'Dombo!'

At last! That was his voice! His little brother was there. He was throwing down his weapons, stopping the men in their wild rush and barring their way with outstretched arms. Then he ran towards him and N'Dombo swung him up in the air, and put him down very gently, on his neck. Then N'Dombo stepped forward proudly like a royal elephant carrying a chief.

'N'Dombo! It's our N'Dombo!'

The whole village was shouting his name. They all recognized him. Soon they were helping to pull out the spears that were still sticking into the folds of his thick hide.

Some young men had gone running off towards the huts and came back with tom-toms. The women clapped their hands to the rhythm and the girls started their shrill singing. Soon masked dancers were stamping on the hard ground with their bare feet, shaking their rattling necklaces and all the tiny bells they wore round their wrists and ankles.

'N'Dombo! N'Dombo has come back!'

They made way for him and he stepped delicately between the mud huts, making sure that there was room to put his round feet down.

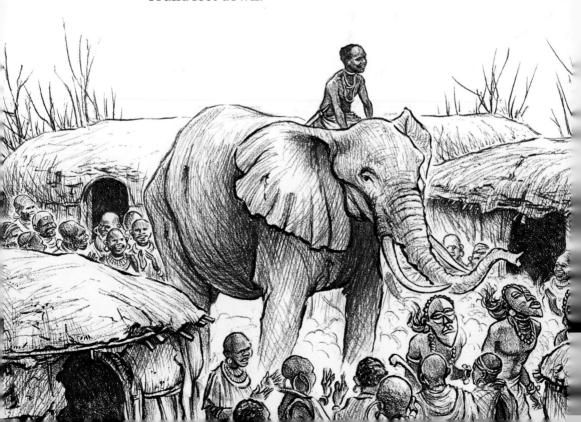

The village was thrilled. They went on beating the tom-toms all night and they danced in gratitude to bush and beast for sending them this messenger – reminding them that the animal kingdom was the finest in the world to live in. This village, after all, was just one among thousands scattered over the Rift; well might they feel proud to enjoy the friendship of the elephants.

The villagers did not go to sleep until morning, and the sun was already high in the sky when they woke. On the other side of the field they found a round patch of flattened grass where N'Dombo the elephant had slept. A smaller hollow, between where his legs had been, showed Wanga's bed.

But neither N'Dombo nor Wanga was there now. They had evidently gone off together, and indeed, at this moment, N'Dombo was completing his mission. He was taking the boy, whom he had come all this way to find, back with him to the green forest kingdom where his tribe was awaiting his return.

Through walls of tall grass in the valley and dense tangles of creepers and undergrowth, N'Dombo carried his little brother on a long, dream-like ride to the mysterious elephant kingdom of which he had told him.

Back in the village, when the elders were told that the elephant had gone off with Wanga into the bush, they only said:

'Wanga's been chosen. That is fair. He was the proudest and bravest, of our young men.'

No one worried about him. The bush would send him back to the village in its own good time.

And this was what Wanga thought too as he rode on N'Dombo's neck along the vast forest's winding trails.

'Where are you taking me, elephant brother?'

The grey trunk twisted back till it was round Wanga's shoulders and gently pushed him forward into a lying position so that they could pass under the low roof of branches which might hurt him.

'Where are you taking me, N'Dombo?'

As he went along N'Dombo picked wild berries and fruit from the bushes for Wanga, choosing those he knew he liked best.

At night Wanga lay with his head on his arms on

N'Dombo's neck and slept. And N'Dombo stuck his huge ears back to his shoulders and held Wanga's long legs safe and firm.

They were approaching the gates of the kingdom along the bottom of the valley. The elephant sentinels posted there saw them coming and hurried back to where the huge herd was waiting.

'It's N'Dombo back again.'

And not alone!

'N'Dombo has brought his brother . . .'

The sun was rising. Wanga woke up. N'Dombo was going at a gentle walking pace over the close-cropped grass.

Then suddenly Wanga caught sight of the enormous herd of wild elephants in the middle of the clearing. There were more than a hundred of them packed close. They were trampling and hammering the ground, as if they were ready to charge, but all the time, as N'Dombo came nearer, they were stepping back to make way and let him into the circle; then they closed in again behind him.

N'Dombo stopped. Then very gently he put Wanga down in the grass at the feet of the ancient noble elders of the herd, the same two great bull elephants who had accompanied him to the edge of the forest. This small figure before them was the man he had been all the way to the plains of the Rift to find.

And now N'Dombo remembered the language used between man and his domestic animals and he made Wanga understand what they wanted him to do.

The elephants stepped back and Wanga saw that they had been hiding a massive elephant lying sprawled on the ground as still as a rock. This was their chief. His head was held up because, in his fall, he had stuck his gigantic tusks into the earth. The boy saw that the elephant was wounded; a stream of blood down his shoulders had congealed into a crust of foul mud, and a little red spring still gushed up behind his neck where an iron spear-head jutted from a gaping wound.

This weapon must have fallen upon the old leader from a trap – one of those traps hunters set with a very heavy iron spear suspended from a forked branch so that it drops with tremendous force when the trap is sprung. The point pierces right to the heart and stays lodged in the flesh because of the hooked barbs on it.

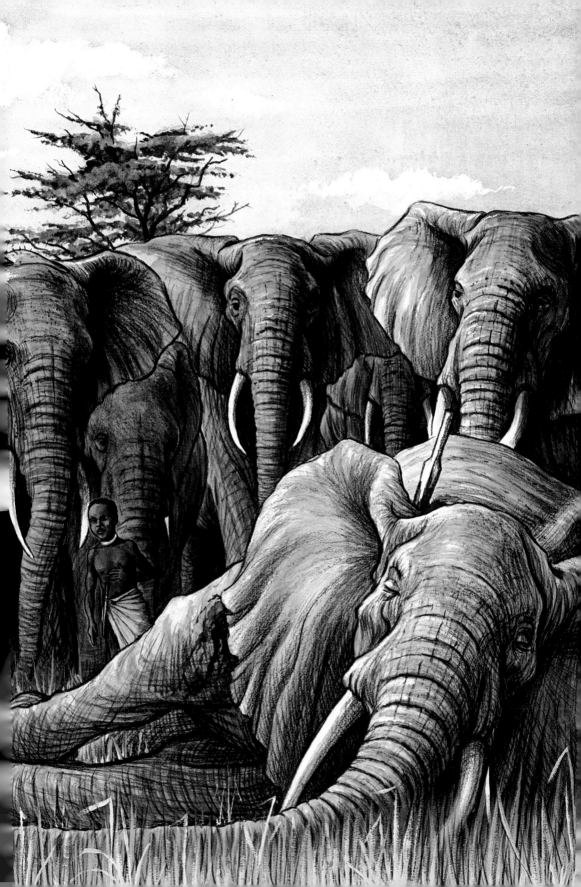

Wanga took his dagger out of its sheath.

Lion, leopard, and panther came down to the foot of the hills to watch from behind the bushes ... the monkeys in the tree-tops looked on – the whole bush was watching the boy from the Tenga country.

Wanga took his dagger and cut all the pieces of red flesh round the spear hooks. Then he spoke to N'Dombo and helped him to get a grip of the great length of iron sticking from the wound so that he could pull it out. Blood spurted out.

Then the great bulls of the tribe came up to their chief. With their tusks they lifted him on to his feet and two of them stood crushed up against him, one on each side to hold him up. Thus their shoulders held him like a vice, and, with their trunks twisted round his tusk to support his drooping head, they managed to hold it up with all its weight of ivory.

The rest of the elephants fell in behind this group, and slowly the procession started off through the long grass.

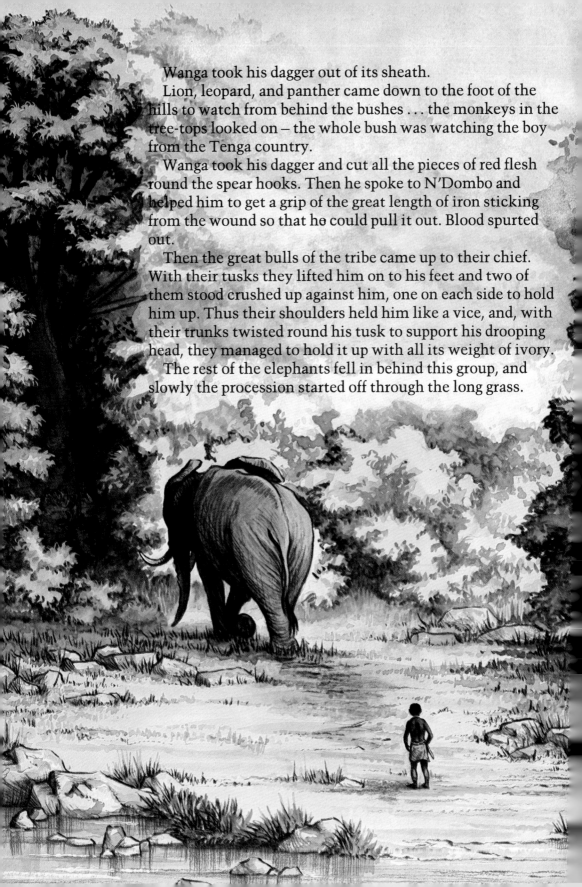

Wanga watched it disappear between the hills. Soon he was alone in the empty valley. Only N'Dombo remained with him. He put his trunk round the boy's waist and lifted him on to his back. Then, stepping out with that long stride of his, he started back through the forest.

Wanga slept through the return journey; the ride through the forest was like a dream. He woke up as N'Dombo halted at the river which wound through the valley of the Rift on its way to Tenga village.

The elephant went down on his knees and took his little brother in his trunk, brought him close to one shining eye and gazed at him, then to the hollow of his huge ear so that Wanga could pour the sweet honey of words into it.

'Up you get, N'Dombo!'

Wanga made his friend get up. Then he took the tip of his trunk in the palm of his hand so as to put him back on the forest path which would lead him home to his wild life – where he belonged.

The docile N'Dombo turned and they walked together past the bushes which had been their playground in the old days.

'Go now, N'Dombo, go back,' Wanga's voice was saying.

'Come, N'Dombo, come,' said the bush, with the voice of the forest.

N'Dombo stood rocking from side to side. He took a step towards the plain and the village, then towards the wood. He did not know which way to go.

'Get along, N'Dombo!'

They both spoke to him as if he were a real animal, the bush and the boy. Both seemed to think that N'Dombo had grown up and had become a proper elephant – and that he ought to go back to his animal life for good.

'Get along now, N'Dombo . . .'

The animal still hesitated. Then, with his trunk hanging down and his tusks low, he turned away at last and plunged into the forest.

René Guillot

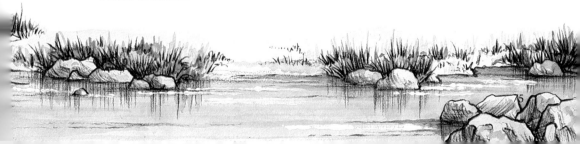

Elephant Song

On the weeping forest, under the evening wind,
Black night has lain down joyfully,
In the sky the stars have fled, trembling,
Fireflies that shine vaguely and go out.
Up there, the moon is dark, its white light has gone out.
The spirits are wandering.
Elephant hunter, take your bow!

Chorus:
    Elephant hunter, take your bow!

In the frightened forest the tree sleeps, leaves are dead.
Monkeys have shut their eyes, hanging high in the branches,
Antelopes slip along with silent steps,
Crop the fresh grass, prick up their ears, intent,
Raise their heads and listen, startled.
The cicada falls silent, shutting in its rasping song.
Elephant hunter, take your bow!

Chorus:
    Elephant hunter, take your bow!

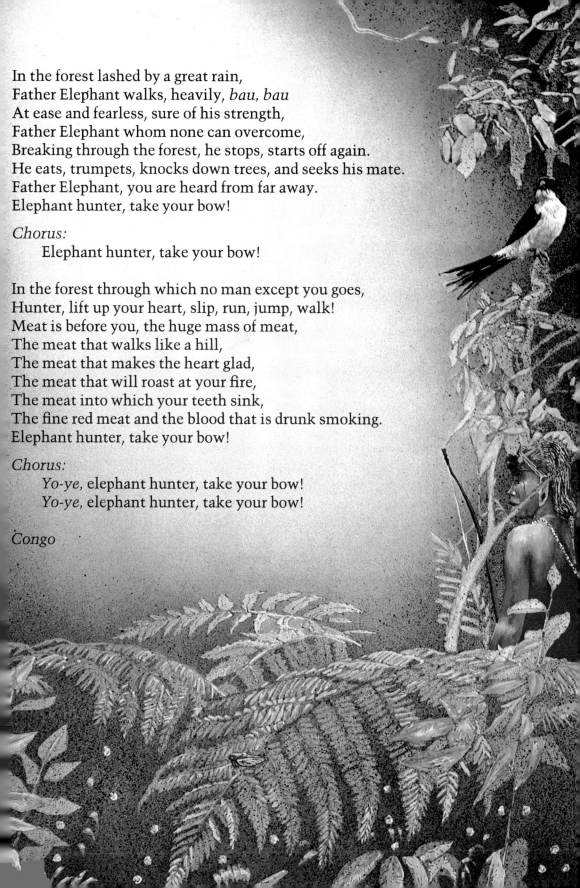

In the forest lashed by a great rain,
Father Elephant walks, heavily, *bau, bau*
At ease and fearless, sure of his strength,
Father Elephant whom none can overcome,
Breaking through the forest, he stops, starts off again.
He eats, trumpets, knocks down trees, and seeks his mate.
Father Elephant, you are heard from far away.
Elephant hunter, take your bow!

Chorus:
    Elephant hunter, take your bow!

In the forest through which no man except you goes,
Hunter, lift up your heart, slip, run, jump, walk!
Meat is before you, the huge mass of meat,
The meat that walks like a hill,
The meat that makes the heart glad,
The meat that will roast at your fire,
The meat into which your teeth sink,
The fine red meat and the blood that is drunk smoking.
Elephant hunter, take your bow!

Chorus:
    Yo-ye, elephant hunter, take your bow!
    Yo-ye, elephant hunter, take your bow!

Congo

Elephant Hunt

I was hunting through very thick forest at the time, camping rough, with only an African guide and a couple of bearers. Time was short because money was running out, but I was determined to get that hundred-pounder before I went much further. Well, on this particular morning we came across the tracks of a small breeding herd, cows and calves, and a little farther on the fresh tracks of two bull elephants, moving on their own. Presently the track of the cows went right across that of the bulls, from left to right, and I thought, 'Thank God the cows and calves are out of the way, so that I can follow up the bulls and get a look at their tusks.' After a little while, edging up very cautiously through the trees, I heard the sound of elephant not far ahead; I had very sharp hearing in those days, not like now. I took my rifle – we had only the one – and sent back my people a little way, as was my custom. Almost at once I heard the sound of a single shot, a muzzle-loader, and asked the guide if he thought there were any Africans near by who might be taking a crack at the elephant. He said he thought it improbable; we were near the edge of the forest, with open plain beyond, and he thought it likely that someone was taking a shot at a water-buck. This seemed a reasonable explanation, and I went on alone.

Presently I came to a small clearing, about six paces across, and partly concealed in the bushes on the other side of it were my two elephants. The first was facing me, the whole of the head and forepart rising out of the scrub; of the other I could see only a patch of hide, and didn't know what part of the animal I was looking at. As I could see at once, the elephant facing me was very, very angry. (I discovered later, these were two of the cows, not bulls at all, and what had annoyed her was undoubtedly that shot.) She was standing with her ears and tail up, ominously swinging her head from side to side. The tusks, as I saw to my disappointment, were very small, so I ran a little way across the clearing to try and get a better view of the other animal.

It was a very foolish thing to do, as were all my actions on this particular occasion. I was asking for it. The next thing I saw, out of the tail of my eye, was the first elephant coming purposefully towards me. I turned and fired a shot at the head

– I was very cocky in those days and thought I could stop any elephant with a single shot. She came on without a pause, and before I could fire again she was very close indeed. It's usual, you know, for a charging elephant to come at you with the head lowered and the chin stretched out, tusks advancing close to the ground, like a cow-catcher. I had barely time to fire a shot at the face, with the animal still coming, and did the only thing possible – turned and made a flying dive for the bush. Of course the inevitable happened; I tripped my foot

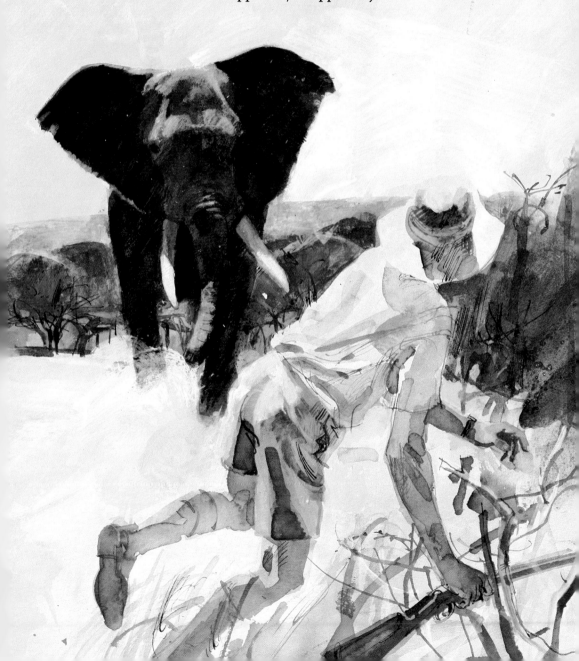

over a branch and fell flat on my face. I lay still, praying that she'd miss the target and wouldn't find me. There was an extraordinary pause. The next thing I knew was a crash of twigs all round and the tusks appeared a foot or so in front of my head, digging up the ground. Looking up I saw a grey chin hanging above me, and knew that I couldn't get away. This was a moment that ought to have inspired the maximum of fear, but I distinctly remember thinking, almost with detachment, 'Now I shall never get that hundred-pounder that I was working so hard for.' The next feeling was also quite dull and detached, as though all this were happening to somebody else. I thought, 'I've been asking for this for quite a long time, and now it looks as though I've got it.' I did not feel at all afraid.

The next thing was that the tusks had disappeared and

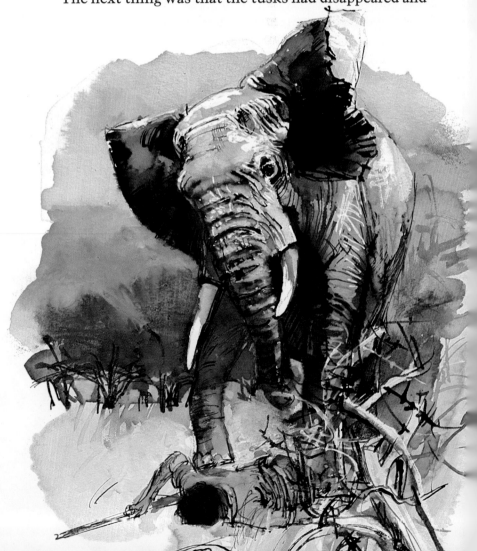

something very heavy came down between my shoulders and scraped me violently backwards along the ground. The pressure was heavy, so that I had difficulty in breathing, but I felt no pain. The next thing she did was to start kicking me about between her fore and hind feet; I can distinctly remember trying to roll out of the way, but with about the third blow I passed out and I've no idea what happened after that.

When I came round I was lying on my face in a different part of the clearing, some distance from the spot where the elephant had caught me. I couldn't see out of one eye; I was in no pain but I felt deathly ill, and could still hear the elephant rumbling very near. There was nothing to do but to go on lying there, hoping that the elephant would call it a day and not bother any more about me. Their fits of temper are short, as a general rule. But I lay for a very long time while nothing happened, and presently it seemed to me that the rumbling was farther off. I started to turn my head very slowly, moving it as slowly, I hoped, as the hands of a clock, and at last I could see that the clearing was trampled and empty; the elephant had disappeared, though I could still hear her in the bushes at a little distance.

I cautiously wiped my eye, which I thought was burst, and found it was not my blood but hers which had been blinding me. I shook my limbs one by one and found nothing broken, though my head felt funny; one of her feet had caught me a blow on the ear which I afterwards found had permanently damaged my hearing. I couldn't walk, but I could crawl; my feet were tangled up in my shorts, which had been pulled very nearly off; I soon got out of those, I can tell you. I managed to get into the bushes, and there my Africans – who were quite unarmed and very near, I take off my hat to them – gathered me up and supported me back to camp.

It took a long time, and all that day and the next I felt frightfully ill. I was sick and faint and very tired. Now that it was all over I had spasms of sweating fear; it kept coming over me in waves. And then of course there were the nightmares. Very bad they were. Oh, shocking. But there it is; in this whole business the *real* pleasure, what one calls the excitement, is simply another name for, another phase of fear. Without the fear one wouldn't be able to enjoy it. Odd, isn't it?

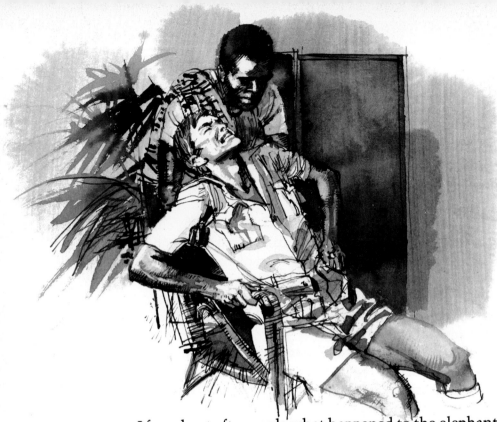

I found out afterwards what happened to the elephant. My
rifle had been left in the clearing, and as it was the only one I
had it had got to be retrieved. My gunbearer had managed to
borrow a rifle from somewhere, and as I couldn't go myself I
sent him back next day to look for mine. Though nothing was
broken I was black and blue and stiff as a board; oh yes, quite
literally. When I wanted to sit up I had to be levered up in one
piece, like a plank. Stiff as hell I was for days; couldn't walk. I
gave my man strict instructions to be careful; if he so much
as heard elephant he was to come straight back, and wait till
the coast was clear.

Well, he went off, and after a time I heard a single shot, and
then silence. I suffered considerable anxiety, you can
imagine; he might have been injured or killed, and there was I
helpless, able to do nothing. But he came back in the evening
all right, complete with my hat and rifle and the elephant's
tusks. My first bullet, he'd found, had passed right through
the head, and my second through the thick part of the trunk
and below the brain. There was blood all over the shop, and
she'd torn up the ground with her tusks in three places.

Ionides

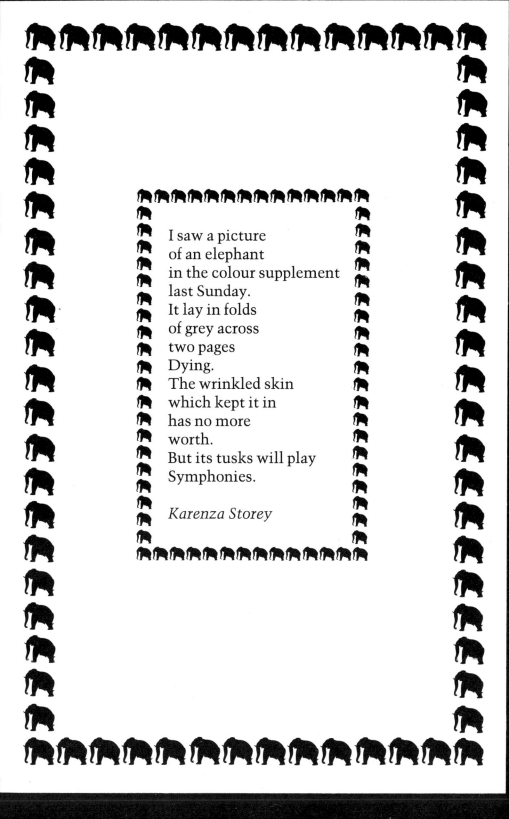

I saw a picture
of an elephant
in the colour supplement
last Sunday.
It lay in folds
of grey across
two pages
Dying.
The wrinkled skin
which kept it in
has no more
worth.
But its tusks will play
Symphonies.

Karenza Storey

Toomai and the Elephant Dance

Little Toomai slept for some time, and when he waked it was brilliant moonlight, and Kala Nag was still standing up with his ears cocked. Little Toomai turned, rustling in the fodder, and watched the curve of his big back against half the stars in heaven; and while he watched he heard, so far away that it sounded no more than a pinhole of noise pricked through the stillness, the 'hoot-toot' of a wild elephant.

All the elephants in the lines jumped up as if they had been shot, and their grunts at last waked the sleeping mahouts, and they came out and drove in the picket-pegs with big mallets, and tightened this rope and knotted that till all was quiet. One new elephant had nearly grubbed up his picket, and Big Toomai took off Kala Nag's leg-chain and shackled that elephant fore-foot to hind-foot, but slipped a loop of grass-string round Kala Nag's leg, and told him to remember that he was tied fast. He knew that he and his father and his grandfather had done the very same thing hundreds of times before. Kala Nag did not answer to the order by gurgling, as he usually did. He stood still, looking out across the moonlight, his head a little raised, and his ears spread like fans, up to the great folds of the Garo hills.

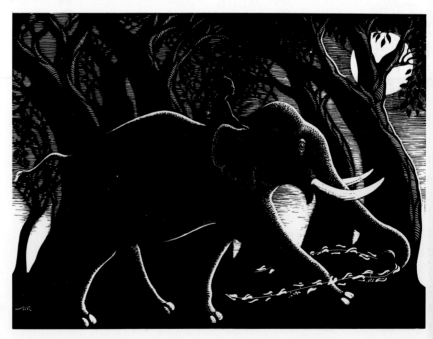

'Look to him if he grows restless in the night,' said Big Toomai to Little Toomai, and he went into the hut and slept. Little Toomai was just going to sleep, too, when he heard the coir string snap with a little 'tang,' and Kala Nag rolled out of his pickets as slowly and as silently as a cloud rolls out of the mouth of a valley. Little Toomai pattered after him, barefooted, down the road in the moonlight, calling under his breath, 'Kala Nag! Kala Nag! Take me with you, O Kala Nag!' The elephant turned without a sound, took three strides back to the boy in the moonlight, put down his trunk, swung him up to his neck, and almost before Little Toomai had settled his knees slipped into the forest.

There was one blast of furious trumpeting from the lines, and then the silence shut down on everything, and Kala Nag began to move. Sometimes a tuft of high grass washed along his sides as a wave washes along the sides of a ship, and sometimes a cluster of wild-pepper vines would scrape along his back, or a bamboo would creak where his shoulder touched it; but between those times he moved absolutely without any sound, drifting through the thick Garo forest as though it had been smoke. He was going uphill, but though Little Toomai watched the stars in the rifts of the trees, he could not tell in what direction.

Then Kala Nag reached the crest of the ascent and stopped for a minute, and Little Toomai could see the tops of the trees lying all speckled and furry under the moonlight for miles and miles, and the blue-white mist over the river in the hollow. Toomai leaned forward and looked, and he felt that the forest was awake below him – awake and alive and crowded. A big brown fruit-eating bat brushed past his ear; a porcupine's quills rattled in the thicket; and in the darkness between the tree-stems he heard a hog-bear digging hard in the moist, warm earth, and snuffing as it digged.

Then the branches closed over his head again, and Kala Nag began to go slowly down into the valley – not quietly this time, but as a runaway gun goes down a steep bank – in one rush. The huge limbs moved as steadily as pistons, eight feet to each stride, and the wrinkled skin of the elbow-points rustled. The undergrowth on either side of him ripped with a noise like torn canvas, and the saplings that he heaved away right and left with his shoulders sprang back again, and banged him on the flank, and great trails of creepers, all matted together, hung from his tusks as he threw his head from side to side and ploughed out his pathway. Then Little Toomai laid himself down close to the great neck, lest a swinging bough should sweep him to the ground, and he wished that he were back in the lines again.

The grass began to get squashy, and Kala Nag's feet sucked and squelched as he put them down, and the night mist at the bottom of the valley chilled Little Toomai. There was a splash and a trample, and the rush of running water, and Kala Nag strode through the bed of a river, feeling his way at each step. Above the noise of the water, as it swirled round the elephant's legs, Little Toomai could hear more splashing and some trumpeting both up stream and down – great grunts and angry snortings, and all the mist about him seemed to be full of rolling, wavy shadows.

'*Ai!*' he said, half aloud, his teeth chattering. 'The elephant-folk are out to-night. It *is* the dance, then.'

Kala Nag swashed out of the water, blew his trunk clear, and began another climb; but this time he was not alone, and he had not to make his path. That was made already, six feet

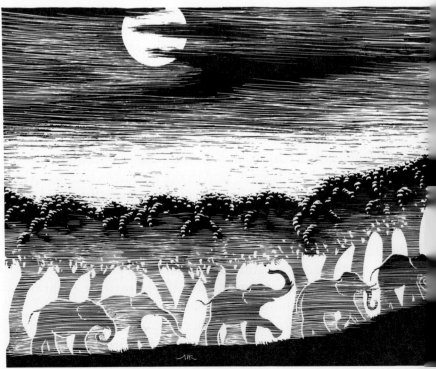

wide, in front of him, where the bent jungle-grass was trying
to recover itself and stand up. Many elephants must have
gone that way only a few minutes before. Little Toomai
looked back, and behind him a great wild tusker, with his
little pig's eyes glowing like hot coals, was just lifting himself
out of the misty river. Then the trees closed up again, and
they went on and up, with trumpetings and crashings, and the
sound of breaking branches on every side of them.

At last Kala Nag stood still between two tree-trunks at the
very top of the hill. They were part of a circle of trees that
grew round an irregular space of some three or four acres, and
in all that space, as Little Toomai could see, the ground had
been trampled down as hard as a brick floor. Some trees grew
in the centre of the clearing, but their bark was rubbed away,
and the white wood beneath showed all shiny and polished in
the patches of moonlight. There were creepers hanging from
the upper branches, and the bells of the flowers of the
creepers, great waxy white things like convolvuluses, hung
down fast asleep; but within the limits of the clearing there
was not a single blade of green – nothing but the trampled
earth.

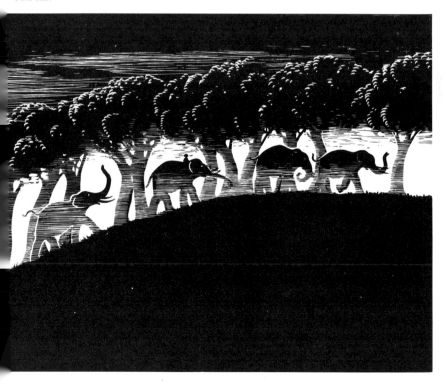

The moonlight showed it all iron-grey, except where some elephants stood upon it, and their shadows were inky black. Little Toomai looked, holding his breath, with his eyes starting out of his head, and as he looked, more and more and more elephants swung out into the open from between the tree-trunks. Little Toomai could count only up to ten, and he counted again and again on his fingers till he lost count of the tens, and his head began to swim. Outside the clearing he could hear them crashing in the undergrowth as they worked their way up the hillside; but as soon as they were within the circle of the tree-trunks they moved like ghosts.

There were white-tusked wild males, with fallen leaves and nuts and twigs lying in the wrinkles of their necks and the folds of their ears; fat, slow-footed she-elephants, with restless little pinky-black calves only three or four feet high running under their stomachs; young elephants with their tusks just beginning to show, and very proud of them; lanky, scraggy old-maid elephants, with their hollow, anxious faces, and trunks like rough bark; savage old bull-elephants, scarred from shoulder to flank with great weals and cuts of bygone fights, and the caked dirt of their solitary mud-baths dropping from their shoulders; and there was one with a broken tusk and the marks of the full-stroke, the terrible drawing scrape, of a tiger's claws on his side.

They were standing head to head, or walking to and fro across the ground in couples, or rocking and swaying all by themselves – scores and scores of elephants.

Toomai knew that, so long as he lay still on Kala Nag's neck, nothing would happen to him; for even in the rush and scramble of a Keddah-drive a wild elephant does not reach up with his trunk and drag a man off the neck of a tame elephant; and these elephants were not thinking of men that night. Once they started and put their ears forward when they heard the chinking of a leg-iron in the forest, but it was Pudmini, Petersen Sahib's pet elephant, her chain snapped short off, grunting, snuffling up the hillside. She must have broken her pickets, and come straight from Petersen Sahib's camp; and Little Toomai saw another elephant, one that he did not know, with deep rope-galls on his back and breast. He, too, must have run away from some camp in the hills about.

At last there was no sound of any more elephants moving

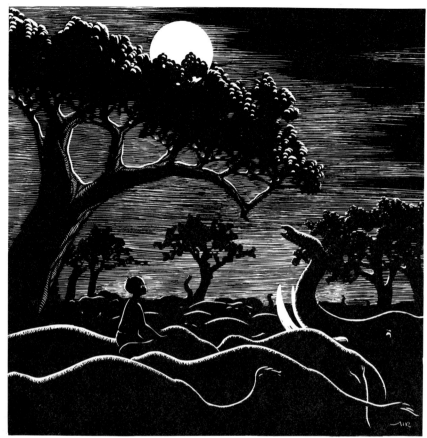

in the forest, and Kala Nag rolled out from his station between the trees and went into the middle of the crowd, clucking and gurgling, and all the elephants began to talk in their own tongue, and to move about.

Still lying down, Little Toomai looked down upon scores and scores of broad backs, and wagging ears, and tossing trunks, and little rolling eyes. He heard the click of tusks as they crossed other tusks by accident, and the dry rustle of trunks twined together, and the chafing of enormous sides and shoulders in the crowd, and the incessant flick and *hissh* of the great tails. Then a cloud came over the moon, and he sat in black darkness; but the quiet, steady hustling and pushing and gurgling went on just the same. He knew that there were elephants all round Kala Nag, and that there was no chance of backing him out of the assembly; so he set his teeth and shivered. In a Keddah at least there was torch-light and shouting, but here he was all alone in the dark, and once a trunk came up and touched him on the knee.

Then an elephant trumpeted, and they all took it up for five or ten terrible seconds. The dew from the trees above spattered down like rain on the unseen backs, and a dull booming noise began, not very loud at first, and Little Toomai could not tell what it was; but it grew and grew, and Kala Nag lifted up one fore-foot and then the other, and brought them down on the ground – one-two, one-two, as steadily as trip-hammers. The elephants were stamping all together now, and it sounded like a war-drum beaten at the mouth of a cave. The dew fell from the trees till there was no more left to fall, and the booming went on, and the ground rocked and shivered, and Little Toomai put his hands up to his ears to shut out the sound. But it was all one gigantic jar that ran through him – this stamp of hundreds of heavy feet on the raw earth. Once or twice he could feel Kala Nag and all the others surge forward a few strides, and the thumping would change to the crushing sound of juicy green things being bruised, but in a minute or two the boom of feet on hard earth began again. A tree was creaking and groaning somewhere near him. He put out his arm and felt the bark, but Kala Nag moved forward, still tramping, and he could not tell where he was in the clearing. There was no sound from the elephants, except once, when two or three little calves squeaked together. Then he heard a thump and a shuffle, and the booming went on. It must have lasted fully two hours, and Little Toomai ached in every nerve; but he knew by the smell of the night air that the dawn was coming.

The morning broke in one sheet of pale yellow behind the green hills, and the booming stopped with the first ray, as though the light had been an order. Before Little Toomai had got the ringing out of his head, before even he had shifted his position, there was not an elephant in sight except Kala Nag, Pudmini, and the elephant with the rope-galls, and there was neither sign nor rustle nor whisper down the hillsides to show where the others had gone.

Little Toomai stared again and again. The clearing, as he remembered it, had grown in the night. More trees stood in the middle of it, but the undergrowth and the jungle-grass at the sides had been rolled back. Little Toomai stared once more. Now he understood the trampling. The elephants had stamped out more room – had stamped the thick grass and

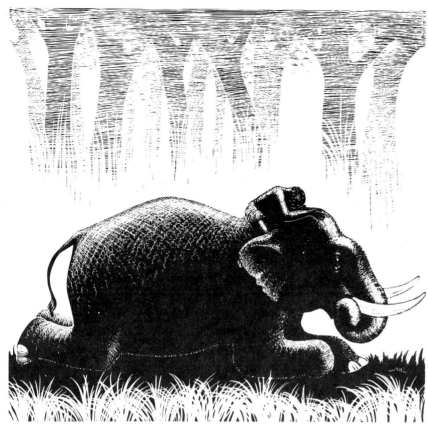

juicy cane to trash, the trash into slivers, the slivers into tiny fibres, and the fibres into hard earth.

'Wah!' said Little Toomai, and his eyes were very heavy. 'Kala Nag, my lord, let us keep by Pudmini and go to Petersen Sahib's camp, or I shall drop from thy neck.'

The third elephant watched the two go away, snorted, wheeled round, and took his own path.

Two hours later, as Petersen Sahib was eating early breakfast, the elephants, who had been double-chained that night, began to trumpet, and Pudmini, mired to the shoulders, with Kala Nag, very foot-sore, shambled into the camp.

Little Toomai's face was grey and pinched, and his hair was full of leaves and drenched with dew; but he tried to salute Petersen Sahib, and cried faintly: 'The dance – the elephant-dance! I have seen it, and – I die!' As Kala Nag sat down, he slid off his neck in a dead faint.

Rudyard Kipling

The Elephants' Graveyard

As Sindbad was returning to Baghdad after a voyage to the King of Serendib his ship was attacked by pirates. He was captured, taken to a lonely island and sold as a slave. The rich merchant who bought him treated him well. One day he asked Sindbad if he knew how to use a bow and arrow.

'I learned how to shoot with them as a young man,' I said, 'and I've not yet forgotten.'

He gave me a bow and arrows and told me to mount behind him on his elephant. We travelled to a huge forest several hours' journey away from the town and stopped at last by a great tree well inside the forest.

'Climb up there,' he said, 'and shoot the elephants that pass underneath. The forest is full of them. If you manage to kill any, come and tell me.'

He gave me food and water and then went back to the town. I stayed up the tree all night, watching and waiting. No elephants came.

As the sun rose next morning a large number of elephants appeared. I shot at them and when at last one fell the others hurried away. My master was delighted with my success and together we dug a hole and buried the dead elephant. He intended to let it rot and then take the tusks and sell them.

In the next two months I killed an elephant every day, sometimes shooting from one tree, sometimes from another. Then, one morning, it was different. The elephants stopped and turned towards the tree in which I was hiding. They came up to it trumpeting loudly and soon the tree was surrounded by more elephants than I had ever seen before. The ground shook beneath them and the air was torn apart by their noise. Countless trunks were aimed at me. I tried to keep still, but I was shaking so much I couldn't even keep hold of my weapons.

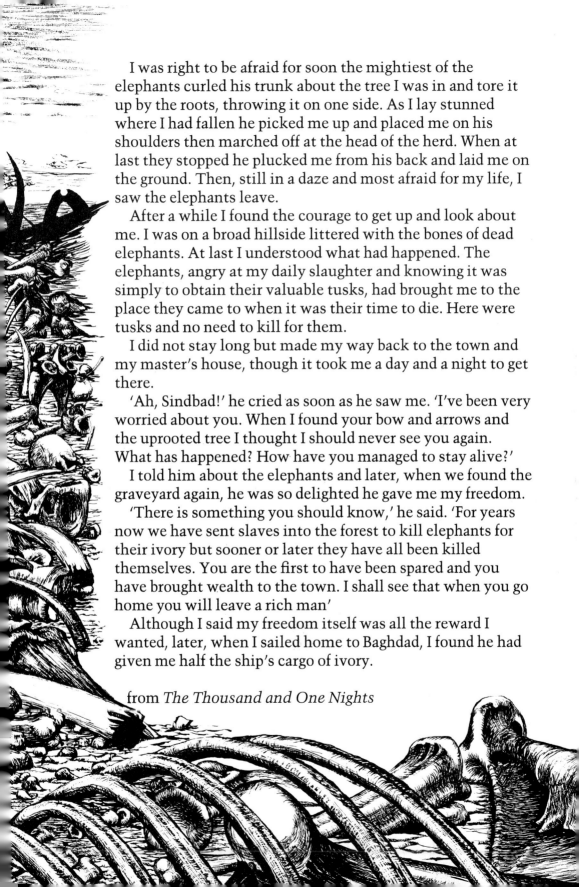

I was right to be afraid for soon the mightiest of the elephants curled his trunk about the tree I was in and tore it up by the roots, throwing it on one side. As I lay stunned where I had fallen he picked me up and placed me on his shoulders then marched off at the head of the herd. When at last they stopped he plucked me from his back and laid me on the ground. Then, still in a daze and most afraid for my life, I saw the elephants leave.

After a while I found the courage to get up and look about me. I was on a broad hillside littered with the bones of dead elephants. At last I understood what had happened. The elephants, angry at my daily slaughter and knowing it was simply to obtain their valuable tusks, had brought me to the place they came to when it was their time to die. Here were tusks and no need to kill for them.

I did not stay long but made my way back to the town and my master's house, though it took me a day and a night to get there.

'Ah, Sindbad!' he cried as soon as he saw me. 'I've been very worried about you. When I found your bow and arrows and the uprooted tree I thought I should never see you again. What has happened? How have you managed to stay alive?'

I told him about the elephants and later, when we found the graveyard again, he was so delighted he gave me my freedom.

'There is something you should know,' he said. 'For years now we have sent slaves into the forest to kill elephants for their ivory but sooner or later they have all been killed themselves. You are the first to have been spared and you have brought wealth to the town. I shall see that when you go home you will leave a rich man'

Although I said my freedom itself was all the reward I wanted, later, when I sailed home to Baghdad, I found he had given me half the ship's cargo of ivory.

from *The Thousand and One Nights*

One elephant gets in the way of lots of people,
Two elephants get in the way of a lot more;
Three elephants get in the way of lots of people,
Four elephants get in the way of a lot more;
Five elephants get in the way of lots of people,
Six elephants get in the way of a lot more;

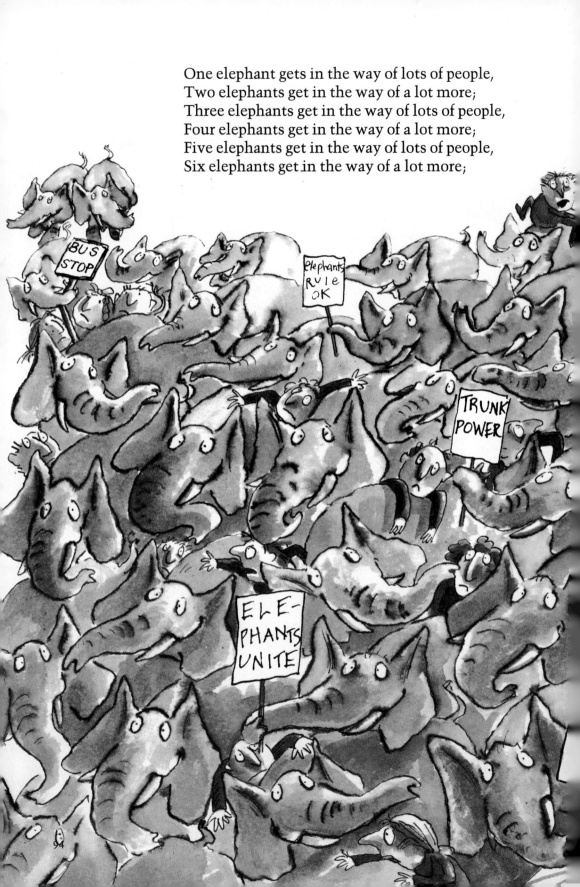

Seven elephants get in the way of lots of people,
Eight elephants get in the way of a lot more;
Nine elephants get in the way of lots of people,
Ten elephants get in the way of a lot more;
Eleven . . . (and so on).

Brazil

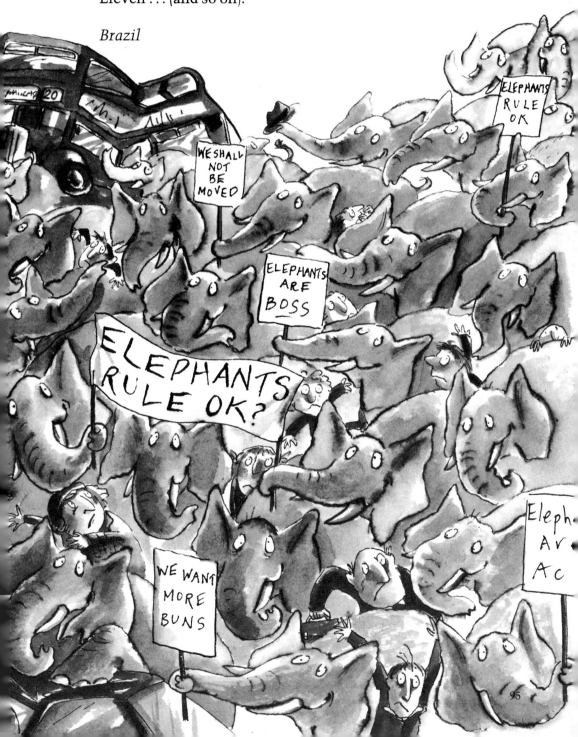

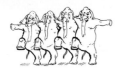

Acknowledgements

Thanks are due to the following for permission to reprint copyright material.

PATRICIA ADAMS: from 'The Elephant and the Beetle', first published in the New South Wales Department of Education's School Magazine. HILAIRE BELLOC: 'The Elephant' from *The Bad Child's Book of Beasts*. Reprinted by permission of Gerald Duckworth & Co. Ltd. A. W. CARDINALL: Adaptation of 'Elephant and Anansi' from pp. 157–161 of *Tales Told in Togoland* (1931; Oxford Reprint 1970) by permission of the International African Institute. I. & O. DOUGLAS-HAMILTON: from *Among the Elephants*. Reprinted by permission of Collins, Publishers. BERNHARD GRZIMEK: from *Among the Animals of Africa*. Reprinted by permission of Collins, Publishers. RENÉ GUILLOT: 'N'dombo the Elephant', adapted from *The Animal Kingdom* by René Guillot, translated by Gwen Marsh © OUP 1957. Reprinted by permission of Oxford University Press. A. E. HOUSMAN: 'The Elephant, or the Force of Habit'. Reprinted by permission of The Society of Authors as the literary representative of the Estate of A. E. Housman, and Jonathan Cape Ltd., publishers of A. E. H. by Laurence Housman. TED HUGHES: 'How the Elephant Became' from *How the Whale Became and Other Stories*. Reprinted by permission of Faber and Faber Ltd. JEAN KENNEDY: 'Little Chow Weighs An Elephant', A Folk Tale of China retold by Jean Kennedy and first published in *Cricket*, Vol. 1, No. 10, July 1975. RUDYARD KIPLING: 'Tha' from 'How Fear Became' from *The Second Jungle Book*; extract from 'The Elephant's Child' from *The Just So Stories*; and extract from 'Toomai of the Elephants' from *The Jungle Book*. Reprinted by permission of A. P. Watt Ltd., on behalf of the National Trust and Macmillan London Ltd. MARGARET LANE: 'Elephant Hunt' from *Life With Ionides*, pp. 93–97. Reprinted by permission of Hamish Hamilton Ltd. OXFORD UNIVERSITY PRESS, INDIA: for permission to reprint 'The Elephant' from *Stories from India*, Book 1. JEROME ROTHENBERG: 'Elephant' from the Yoruba, in *Technicians of the Sacred* by Jerome Rothenberg (Doubleday 1968/Anchor Books 1969). CARL SANDBURG: 'Elephants are Different to Different People' from *The Complete Poems of Carl Sandburg*. Copyright 1950 by Carl Sandburg, renewed 1978 by Margaret Sandburg, Helga Sandburg Crile and Janet Sandburg. Reprinted by permission of Harcourt Brace Jovanovich, Inc. KARENZA STOREY: 'I saw a picture of an elephant . . .'. Reprinted by permission of the author. KATHRYN TAYLOR: 'Tromp! Tromp' from *Big Dipper* (ed. Epstein). Reprinted by permission of Oxford University Press, Australia. E. W. THOMAS: 'A Little Water', adapted from a Kalahari Story, in *Bushman Stories*. Reprinted by permission of Oxford University Press, Southern Africa. J. R. R. TOLKIEN: 'Oliphaunt' from *The Adventures of Tom Bombadil*. Reprinted by permission of George Allen & Unwin (Publishers) Ltd. WILLARD TRASK: 'Elephant Song' from *The Unwritten Song*, Vol. 1, pp. 67–68, edited with translations by Willard R. Trask. Copyright © 1966 by Willard R. Trask. Reprinted by permission of Macmillan Publishing Co., Inc. J. H. WILLIAMS: 'Ma Shwe Saves Her Calf' from *Elephant Bill*. Reprinted by permission of Granada Publishing Ltd. YVONNE WILLIAMS: 'Elephant' was first published in *Impressions*, Summer 1976. Reprinted by permission of High School of Art, Cheetham, Manchester. DAVID HENRY WILSON: from *Elephants Don't Sit on Cars*. Reprinted by permission of Chatto & Windus Ltd., for the author. CARL WITHERS: 'The Elephants' from *I Saw A Rocket Walk A Mile*. Copyright © 1965 by Carl Withers. Reprinted by permission of The Bodley Head and Holt Rinehart and Winston, Publishers.

Cartoons

Sax Cartoon: 'He's in a nasty mood today' from the *Weekend*, Summer Extra No. 10, 1979. Reprinted by permission of Associated Newspapers Group p.l.c. Neville Spearman Ltd: for permission to reproduce two cartoons from Edna Bennett, *The Best Cartoons From France*, Panther Books 1965 © Neville Spearman Ltd., and Arco Publications 1964. Friedrich Karl Waechter: cartoon strip from 'Elephantasies' reproduced by permission of Dobson Books Ltd.

The publishers have made every effort to trace and contact copyright holders, but in some cases without success, and apologize for any infringement of copyright.

Photographs

Ardea 46; Survival Anglia (Lee Lyon) 4/5, 13; Heather Angel 59; Survival Anglia (Dieter Plage) 64.

Illustrations

Illustrations by Allan Curless, Martin Cottam, Priscilla Lamont, Edward McLachlan, John Raynes, Jeroo Roy, Meg Rutherford, Louise Voce, Martin White.